UNCOMMON VOYAGE:

Parenting Children with Special Needs

UNCOMMON VOYAGE:

Parenting Children with Special Needs

A Guidebook

Laura Shapiro Kramer

Cover design by James Rattazzi
Edited by Christine Maloof Corso
Published in 2019 by Blackstone Publishing
ISBN: 978-1-982620-60-8

For my parents
and
for all parents

It matters not how strait the gate,
How charged with punishments the scroll,
I am the master of my fate,
I am the captain of my soul.
—From *"Invictus,"*
by William Ernest Henley

Believe in yourself and be prepared to
work hard.
—From the teachings of
B.K.S. Iyengar

CONTENTS

INTRODUCTION

The sea hath no king but God alone.

—Anonymous

Uncommon Voyage was originally written as a memoir. It was the story of me and of my family after Seth's diagnosis. The book described Seth's development and education and included the story of *my* development and education. It described the person I became as the parent of a special-needs child. My exploration and eventual embrace of solutions in the world of "alternative" medicine were a big part of the story.

With Seth's diagnosis so began my unfurling. The ship I was on was not going on a direct route. I was in uncharted waters with my family—my precious cargo—on board. The only thing to do was to take charge and steer my vessel myself and take on board the best I could find. Eventually I left the safety of the harbor, ventured to another world, changed course, and found help for Seth and meaning for me.

There was nothing to help at first. (There was no internet, no Google.) I did not find a cohesive perspective—relevant personal experience, practical information, and resources—all in one place. Eventually I came to realize that such a thing could only exist if I created it for myself, and I did so by finding people who knew more than I did and combining it with what I knew deep down; by researching, trying things on myself, ultimately having the courage to use what I learned about me for Seth. Life became create and recreate, invent and re-invent.

After the first edition of *Uncommon Voyage* was published, parents reached out to me for support, for direction and ideas, and for a boost. They asked me what to do, what else I knew—I never stopped learning—and I found myself explaining in more detail what I discovered for Seth, how it shaped our family, and how it shaped me. I listened. The more I listened, the more I learned. What I realize is that throughout the journey, the deeper questions about life keep surfacing. Many of the questions I was asking as Seth's mother—a parent of a special-needs child and his sibling—I was asking as a person examining her life.

In this edition of the book, I consider those universal and recurring questions and weave them into a practical guide. I made this edition of *Uncommon Voyage* a vehicle for *your* story, *your* voyage—how you see it, tell it, and are informed by it. I lay the groundwork in a brief narrative that describes my personal journey. I conceived the voyage in nautical terms thinking about a ship's fulcrum—how the shifts in a family's life are like the swinging pieces of a mobile, relocating to attain balance like a vessel rocking on the sea. As changes come along, we continually recalibrate our internal and external compasses to balance and to be able to pivot when necessary.

I developed this guidebook and organized the chapters based on the different aspects of being the parent of a special-needs child. Each chapter offers *Navigation Points* marked by compasses, and lighthouses illuminating *Laura's Insights*.

Navigation Points are tasks to help you chart your course and identify what tools you have and what tools you need.

Laura's Insights are comments offering support. They give context for the endeavor to help you maintain your course.

You decide how far you journey, you determine the pace, and you judge when and where you double back or venture into uncharted waters. Within *Uncommon Voyage* there is an array of resources and experiments to explore. There is a suggested reading list within each chapter, and at the end of the book you will find a glossary, appendices, and additional suggested reading lists. I included a *Ship's Manifest* for handy reference to keep track of who is who. Additional resources—including links to websites and organizations—reside on the Uncommon Voyage web site, and I invite you to join the *Uncommon Voyage* community through Facebook and Twitter to interact with me and with others. I encourage you to ask questions and to share what you know. We learn from one another.

I gave thought to making this book easy to use and read. When deciding on a personal pronoun, rather than switching between "he" and "she" (I found the use of "one" or "they" a bit awkward), I have used "he" throughout this book to reflect my voyage with Seth. I hope that readers with daughters or children of indeterminate gender feel comfortable substituting the pronoun of choice as they read. I researched and chose the font *Georgia* for readability on both paper and screen.

The world of special needs is not a world where we are saved by some ready-made cohesive plan, or even where there is a set destination. The best we can do is catch the waves and go with the flow. Those who head out on an ocean voyage are wise to fortify and provision their ship and map out a general course. I am telling my story and offering navigation to help you discover your own path and to find the support you need for wherever you are on your child's, your family's, your *own* journey.

Uncommon Voyage does not address individual conditions. I am relating to our universal experience. No matter the diagnosis—autism to schizophrenia to cerebral palsy—some things belong to all of us. Shock, ambivalence, chafing between doing too much and doing too little, grief, worry, guilt, living with shattered dreams—we have common experience even within the differences. I hope there is enough here to help you feel less alone while you fight to give your child the best chance at a future of promise and discovery. The miracles are not what you expect but they are there.

Laura Shapiro Kramer
January 2017

LANDMARKS

This book contains multiple links to resources in the form of books and links to web sites. In addition, you will find links to our online community at my web site, uncommonvoyage.com, and on Facebook and Twitter.

You can access an expanded Resource Guide by clicking the link below.

If you are reading a paper version of this book, I invite you to visit the following web site:

http://www.LauraShapiroKramer.com/resources1897/

SHIP'S MANIFEST
A handy guide to recall passengers on the voyage.

In order of appearance

Jay: my husband

Amy: Seth's first pediatric physical therapist

Dr. L: our pediatrician

Annie: my physical therapist

Susan: a pediatric physical therapist recommended by Amy & Annie

Peggy: Seth's occupational therapist

Dr. G: a pediatric orthopedist

Mayra: a part-time helper who provided assistance with Seth

Dr. Daniel Kessler: a pediatrician specializing in developmental disabilities

Charles: a local Feldenkrais teacher

Anat Baniel: a renowned Feldenkrais practitioner, especially with children

Carola Speads: a renowned teacher of body work, especially movement and breathing

Mia Segal: the leader of my Feldenkrais training

Haya: my daughter

Dr. Domenick Masiello: a cranial osteopath and homeopath who treated first me, then Seth and Haya

Dr. Viola Frymann: a cranial osteopath and founder of the internationally-renowned Osteopathic Center for Children in San Diego, recommended to us by Dr Masiello

Peter Springall: Seth's sensory motor learning specialist, recommended by Dr. Frymann

Stoney: a college baseball player and Seth's summer trainer

Carl Stough ("Dr. Breath"): breathing specialist who worked weekly with Seth for ten years

A BRIEF NARRATIVE OF
MY PERSONAL VOYAGE

Jay and I were married for four years when I got pregnant in 1982. Jay is an attorney with a passion for baseball. I was independent producing and had worked on Broadway and in Hollywood. We delayed starting a family while we were trying to establish ourselves. When we did conceive, I was almost thirty-five and healthy. I was careful about what I ate, I exercised regularly, and did not smoke.

A friend recommended her obstetrician-gynecologist and I went to see him. He was charming and confident and, yet appeared slightly cavalier about my pregnancy. I was not entirely comfortable with him but I did not know if it was him or me. I lacked the self-confidence (or the guts) to question or challenge him. He was the one wearing the white coat. Like many of us I came into the doctor-patient relationship believing doctors have the answers. I relied totally on what the doctor said even though his unconditional stance on some aspects of my upcoming delivery caused some doubts; I kept them to myself. After genetic counseling, a few tests, and an amniocentesis, we knew we were expecting a healthy boy. I was having a good pregnancy, feeling well and taking care of myself.

After what was a prolonged night of contractions and pain the birth itself was a nightmare. During labor the doctor left the room only to return hours later to administer Pitocin and disappear again. Seth was born on a labor table in the hospital hallway two weeks after his due date. He aspirated meconium (a word I had never heard until then) and immediately after the delivery he was whisked off to the Neonatal Intensive Care Unit (NICU).

Back in my room, my first visitor was a social worker. The hospital had procedures in place so that she was there to warn me about what I was going to see in the NICU; that Seth would be hooked up to lots of tubes; that he would be in an incubator. I was furious. I did not want to hear anything. I believed I would not be affected by what I would see. I just wanted to see my baby. I rejected her and her attempts to prepare me.

Though Seth weighed over eight pounds, except for feedings he remained in an incubator in the NICU. I made allies of some NICU nurses and they helped me learn to breastfeed. It was not easy but I persevered. For three days I never left his side, defying hospital policies about access.

I could not believe my own transformation. Hours, days, and months earlier, I was willing to go along with whatever the doctor had to say. Now that it was about my child, now that I was a parent, I was standing up to him and to others. Little did I know I was already beginning to grow into the person I eventually became: an advocate for my child.

After the three days, the doctors unplugged the monitors, said Seth was a "champ" and Jay and I took him home; a new family with no hint of anything wrong. Seeing the rocking chair and crib, the nursery full of typical baby stuff, I forgot the nightmare of the delivery; joy buried all thoughts of the recent trauma. Seth was a wonderful, easy baby, so it never occurred to me to worry about the events surrounding his birth. In fact, I was eager to forget them. An alarm bell went off when Seth was five weeks old. However, I did see a boy his age put an object in his mouth: perfect hand/eye coordination like I had never seen Seth do. I stifled the warning. How could there be anything wrong with him?

Seth was born at the time here in the United States when discussion about the positive effects of massage for babies was just beginning. I wanted to take advantage of this trend so when he was just a few weeks old I scheduled an appointment with a massage therapist who worked in the same place where I went swimming.

When she finished the massage, the masseuse startled me by saying, "He's very stiff, and you must stroke his head a lot." She demonstrated a caressing motion across the top of Seth's skull away from his forehead, and went on repeating how stiff he was. I was stunned. I seethed; the gall that anyone dare to diminish my son's obvious perfection. Without letting her see my upset, I dressed Seth and went away.

My reaction was a combination of feeling scared, slightly close minded, and being a neophyte—what did I know about how a baby should *feel?* For me he felt fine. What I saw as an insult to Seth's perfection was actually an expert offering genuine insight and advice. At that point in time I saw only doctors as qualified experts. I discounted the insights of the masseuse.

Four years later when our daughter was born I certainly *felt* the difference. Years after the encounter with the massage therapist I remembered her advice about stroking Seth's skull while I watched a world-renowned doctor do just that. I am ahead of myself. You will learn more as you read on.

Seth grew older. Weeks and months went by and our pediatrician, Dr. L., kept tamping down my fears and anxieties about what I intuited were our son's delays. Seth was ten months old and not yet sitting up, never mind pulling himself to stand. He was not crawling. He was supposed to be ready for a playgroup, but when we explored the options and saw what other children his age were doing—standing, climbing—I knew he could not be a part of it. Something was not right. I had to act.

On a recommendation from a knowledgeable friend, I called a pediatric physical therapist, Amy. She came to the apartment on a Saturday morning and at the end of her session with Seth, she told me, "He has a lot of good movement in him. He needs to be seen by a doctor who knows more than me." She strongly encouraged us to get a neurological evaluation. I was very nervous and kept probing her. Over and over she repeated he had a lot of good movement in him and we should get him looked at by a neurologist.

Even though it was the weekend, I called our pediatrician. She told me, "We may as well get a baseline. After all, he was a meconium baby." This was the first time Dr. L ever mentioned that Seth's aspiration of meconium might be a factor in his development. She recommended a pediatric neurologist and I made an appointment right away.

The doctor interviewed Jay and me about Seth and about the circumstances of his birth (about which I barely remembered anything) and then took Seth into the examination room. After twenty minutes he told us, "Your son will live a normal life. He will eventually walk and he will probably talk and feed and dress himself. But he will never walk normally, and he will not walk for a long time. Your son has mild cerebral palsy."

We were shocked! Stunned. Did someone just punch me in the stomach? The doctor started talking about developmental disabilities and brain scans. When I recovered enough to speak I desperately started to question him. I was hardly prepared to ask anything remotely helpful. He essentially stonewalled us, saying we could try rehabilitation or physical therapy if we wanted, but he did not think anything would really help. He ordered no tests.

Maybe I should have been better prepared to ask questions. I had gone to the consultation not really knowing what a neurologist was and not expecting to hear anything like what he was telling us even though *I knew there was something wrong.* I had been anxious for months owing to intuition and ultimately Amy's observations, yet I never imagined that cerebral palsy would be the diagnosis.

Once the doctor named Seth's disability my world went haywire. My first thoughts were of a boy I knew growing up who had cerebral palsy. I had helped take care of Jimmy over several summers when our families spent time together. I remembered what he was like and it scared me. I barely understood what it was going to mean in Seth's case. Had the label been autism or multiple sclerosis or countless others, I would have been just as ignorant and just as frightened. I felt confused and I felt a chord of primal fear. I tottered between what I hoped for him and every cliché of his disability I could imagine. How was I ever going to look at Seth the same way again?

How would I gauge the dimensions of the problem as it manifested—especially as a new mother and a first-time parent? What did I know about a child's normal development? I had no experience to draw on, no basis for comparison. I wanted reassurance and predictions—to know how it would turn out—and I longed for a set course, a definite route through it all. One thing for sure: whatever else I thought that day, immediately I knew I was the starting point to get the answers and the help Seth needed.

The role I played in the family began emerging right away. It started there and then with Jay in the moment of diagnosis. I was frightened, but the look on Jay's face gave meaning to the word devastation. I reassured him that it would all come out right. I sensed that if I said it would be all right enough times, it would be true, or it would come true. By telling Jay, I was telling myself.

I was responding to my innate optimism, convinced that things could not be as bad as they sounded and that there were remedies, but deep down I was beginning the first phase of being a mother of a special-needs child: finding the fine line between trying to will things to be better and being realistic. I had to do everything I could for Seth while supporting my husband and other family members, "managing" the outside world and my inside world. I remained cheerful—as much as possible—embracing the role that was thrust on me. Optimism was part of it, for Seth, my family, and myself. Optimism and determination a *momentous decision: to use what I did know to find out what I did not know.*

The day of the diagnosis I immediately called two people I knew: the physical therapist, Amy—who had encouraged me to get a neurological evaluation in the first place—and Annie, a physical therapist who was treating me for back pain and some athletic injuries. They both recommended Susan, a pediatric physical therapist who I called right away. She agreed to come to the apartment to see Seth, do an evaluation and prescribe a course of treatment. Susan practiced *neuro-developmental therapy* (NDT), also known as the *Bobath method*. At that point I knew nothing about NDT/the Bobath method, but Susan was the expert with tools. Instantly I turned myself over to her. My solution was to dive into therapy, to get her started. Before I even met her, I felt she was the person who could "fix it."

Susan began coming to the house three times a week. The therapy promised so much that I immediately made her the authority and the barometer of Seth's future. I handed whatever faith I had in myself over to her. I was looking for answers from her and put myself completely in her hands (like Seth who was literally in her hands.) She was positive about Seth's progress. While I relied on Susan to be our captain I asked more questions especially about what else *I* should be doing besides her therapy. Susan admitted she thought Seth needed an occupational thera-pist. Right away on her recommendation we engaged Peggy, an OT who came twice a week. While trained in the NDT method,

Peggy's work was different from Susan's. Her style was a foreshadowing of what we did in the future.

Probing and prodding yielded results. Susan's responses included a referral for a pediatric orthopedist and eventually a pediatric podiatrist. As I continued to grow into my role in our professional relationship, I became increasingly engaged in the process, pursuing options beyond what I was being spoon fed.

The downside of additional input was the fact that professional opinions did not always align. The podiatrist recommended putting Seth in removable casts. (As opposed to braces, these removable casts were heavy plaster casts that covered his legs and feet from the knee down.) The orthopedist said there was no consensus about braces and casts. Add to that while Susan initially said Seth only needed an orthotic, she was now concurring with this more extreme treatment. We went with the casts.

Three months after Seth's initial diagnosis, I stopped and caught my breath and dared to look up cerebral palsy in the dictionary (still no Google!) I got a big jolt when I read, "...a disability resulting from damage to the brain before or during birth and outwardly manifested by muscular incoordination and speech disturbances." Speech! Yikes. No one had ever mentioned anything about speech. I turned to Susan, who recommended a speech therapist. I realized that *no one was going to have all the answers*. I was frantic that time was passing and we had not addressed this important area.

Who was guiding me? Three therapists: one coming two times a week; one coming twice a week and now the speech therapist! And I still felt all alone. How did I keep track and how do I remember the details of Seth's early life and our pursuits on his behalf? I wrote everything down.

How did I have time for this non-stop vigilance and networking in the age before the Internet? I often asked myself: what if I were not self-employed? I was also extremely fortunate to have a part-time helper, Mayra, a young woman who came to work for us a few months after Seth was born. Mayra was often part of Seth's therapy sessions—the six every week—and when I came home from work she would conscientiously recount the sessions and show me what she learned.

Seth was cooperative with Susan and Peggy, the two NDT therapists, but he did not like the speech therapist at all, which in turn affected how I felt about her. After only two weeks of working with Seth, the therapist stunned us by suggesting Seth learn sign language! What? Did that mean he was not going to talk? How did she know? He was only fifteen months old. Was he supposed to be articulating fully comprehensible words?

Frantically I began consulting every baby book I had or could find, looking for guidance in the writings of Penelope Leach and T. Berry Brazelton. Dr. L thought it was premature to make a decision about teaching Seth to sign, but she was unsure. I had no point of reference and was in a complete dither. I had to find someone to help me.

With great effort—including calls, research, and referrals—I found Dr. Daniel Kessler, a developmental disabilities expert, at New York Hospital/Cornell Medical Center. I called to schedule an appointment. The doctor himself picked up the phone and talked to me at length right then. I was in love. Dr. Kessler was just starting his practice. He was not married to any one philosophy plus he was open to working either as a consultant or as Seth's primary care physician. After months of facing mixed messages, differences of opinion, and contradicting forecasts, it felt like I was finally talking to someone who was helping us. Dr. Kessler focused on my son as an individual and not just a diagnosis, and always *included me in the process* by sharing what he was thinking as he developed the ideas for what would most help Seth.

Less than a year later, Dr. Kessler left New York for Phoenix and founded Southwest Human Development. He is now nationally known for his work with children with behavioral and developmental difficulties, particularly on the autism spectrum. Dr. Kessler left me a legacy: he endowed me with my first real sense that I could trust myself. These were my first steps in becoming an advocate. One of my first decisions in this new role was to "stand up to" the speech therapist. Jay concurred that we were not teaching Seth sign language.

Throughout this time, my physical therapist, Annie, was talking to me constantly about the Feldenkrais (FELL-den-krīz) method. I could barely say or spell the word, never mind contemplate jumping into something that sounded so "out there." However, Annie had been my initial referral to our valuable "Captain" Susan, so I already viewed her as a reliable source of information. Afraid of alienating her and wanting to be open minded, I agreed to learn more about this *alternative* method. I had no idea then how important the Feldenkrais work would eventually become.

I heard Anat Baniel's name for the first time in these conversations with Annie about Feldenkrais. Anat was the protégée of founder Moshe Feldenkrais. At that time Anat was teaching and doing this revolutionary work with children and adults in Israel and Canada. I was determined to learn more about the method—I was intrigued—so I scheduled an appointment for Seth with Charles, a local Feldenkrais practitioner.

At our initial meeting, Charles asked a few preliminary questions and spent an hour handling Seth. Seth was comfortable with him because he was already familiar with some of the "moves." Charles was very reassuring. He said Susan was doing everything he himself would do and that his "fantasy" was that Seth would have absolutely no perceptible difficulties. I was thrilled. Charles said that if Seth's feet developed well, there would be no hip problems; I questioned him and learned as he patiently explained the many relationships within the "soma." What he revealed gave me my first true understanding of the body's function and structure. (The foot bone is connected to the ankle bone is connected to the shin bone is connected to the knee bone is connected to the thigh bone is connected to the hip bone.)

At fifteen months, Seth was not standing independently or even pulling himself to stand. Because of this, he especially loved his walker, where he sat in a sling-like seat on wheels. This gave him mobility, allowing him to move from place to place in the apartment like other children his age who were already walking and getting around independently. At the same time, I was aware of some disagreement about walkers.

Peggy, the occupational therapist, was opposed to Seth's using the walker. She believed he should stand only when development allowed for standing or his feet would be compromised. On the other hand, Dr. L had recommended the walker in the first place, and she pooh-poohed Peggy's criticism. Of course we asked "Captain" Susan for her opinion. She had no objections to the walker.

Once again I was faced with making the final decision with conflicting input from experts. Were there two "right" answers? Two "wrong" answers? There was a lot of pressure. It once again fell to me to make the decision, and I simply made a practical one for us at the time: Seth was fifteen months old and getting heavier to carry. The walker made life easier for me.

It was a year after the initial diagnosis and I was confident and hopeful on some days and nervous on others, two emotions snaking through me whether I was awake or asleep. Jay and I were overwhelmed (some would say I was obsessed). Casts and walkers were only two concerns. In addition there were more complex questions about if and when to intervene to help Seth with a task: how much frustration was okay? Plus I was having to learn to be political, balancing our personal and professional relationships with those helping Seth with the life of our family. This was my earliest perception that a mobile is a perfect metaphor for living in relationship to others; the most important aspect is a solid fulcrum—focus on what nourishes the family.

Everything was turned upside down when Seth was two and a half—still wearing the casts—and I had back surgery. It was an extreme step but I could not work to balance our ship until I took care of myself. Annie was continuing to propose alternative techniques to manage pain. She never stopped talking about Feldenkrais and about craniosacral therapy. Seeing that I had an immediate need, she insisted that I get a Feldenkrais practitioner to help me recover. Though I valued the contact to Charles, I made an appointment with the Feldenkrais therapist she recommended because he was a trained physical therapist *and* training rigorously with Anat Baniel.

The Feldenkrais work impacted me immediately: I was always better after the treatments. And I loved it. Although I was the patient, the therapist was persistently curious about Seth; he asked a lot of questions and—like Annie and Charles—he spoke about Anat Baniel. Anat was emerging more and more as the foremost practitioner with children.

A few months later, Anat came to New York to teach a two-week seminar for adults and to give some lectures. I enrolled immediately. In the meantime, I had stayed in touch with Charles, who was prodding me to investigate the work and the classes of Carola Speads. Carola taught "Physical Re-education and Movement" in our neighborhood. It was mainly breath work. I was skeptical but I was in the mood to explore.

Though my days were full with caring for Seth, I saw value in attending these evening classes. In Anat's seminar and Carola's classes, I was introduced to radical therapeutic possibilities that impacted my thinking. The "body work" inspired me. In addition to the effect on my body, *I began learning to hear my inner voice and to trust my intuition.* That intuition was telling me to think of Seth, to connect what I was learning to how it might directly benefit him.

After weeks of revelations, I began to do some "body work" with Seth—the way I was learning in Anat's seminar and Carola's classes. Suddenly, I was at the tiller of the ship. I took charge even though Mayra was still working for us. She had learned from the therapists to do many things with Seth but now I was literally taking him in hand.

So much of my evolution was about peeling away the layers between Seth and me. Engaging therapists and caregivers—no matter how helpful—separated me from Seth. I needed to find a balance between the ways others were helpful and how their presences distanced me from my son. The mobile reacted and shifted as I ensured that fewer layers existed between me and Seth.

We lived a few months with relative equilibrium before a major shift occurred. We received the great news that Anat Baniel was coming to live and work in New York, and she was willing to take Seth on as a patient. Our world shifted to accommodate Anat's demands. Anat saw Seth in her office—not in our home as other practitioners had—and she made a precondition of treating him that we get rid of the other therapists and throw out the casts. She wanted Seth barefoot as much as possible. The walker was an absolute no-no. We were to send Seth to her three times a week: no one else in the room but Seth and Anat. Whoever brought him to sessions waited outside the treatment room. There was no room for argument. Anat had total confidence in herself and she was unequivocal. She made it clear to Seth—and to us—that with her help he would learn to walk. I knew deep down it was true. So did Seth.

From the first moment and the first session with Anat, Seth was changed. He looked and acted differently: stronger and smoother. At three-and-a-half years old, Seth understood that Anat would help him learn to walk, yet at first he struggled with her—it was not all smooth sailing. Seth found that when he did not cooperate with Anat, he was ignored and made to sit in the room until the session was up. He quickly learned to engage and cooperate with Anat. Jay and I noticed visible positive differences in Seth. His upper body dexterity was better; his posture and carriage improved; his eyes were set different in his head.

In the meantime, I struggled to put a public face on the revolutionary work Anat was doing with Seth. Feldenkrais? What would we tell everyone—the family, Dr. L, the therapists, our friends? We were tossing established methods aside for an unpronounceable, untried alternative and I feared they would think we were crazy. Only Peggy the occupational therapist agreed wholeheartedly with what we were doing. Susan and the speech therapist were angry and discouraging.

I was not deterred. Seeing what was happening with Seth and my experience in the two-week seminar with Anat made me curious to learn even more about Feldenkrais. I applied and was accepted to participate in a three-year Feldenkrais training, and enrolled in the first leg with Mia Segal—a student and assistant of Feldenkrais from the 50's. It was exciting to be around other students— physical therapists, Alexander teachers, psychother-apists, musicians, and actors—also training in the Feldenkrais method. I felt much less alone. My respect for them helped me keep faith in the work. It was a long way from Hollywood.

Seth was making noticeable strides: he was feisty and he was stronger. He was talking and his speech was much clearer. We were not not alone in these observations: our parents and the teachers at preschool noted his progress and his growth spurt. Up until this point, our decision about the Feldenkrais work had met with skepticism and glazed stares. Suddenly we were on steadier ground. Within a few months Seth told us, "I am going to learn to walk and Anat is teaching me."

I had faith in the method, but still struggled with the pain of our situation. As part of my routine, I swam at a community center that also housed a nursery school. While riding in the elevator I often overheard parents—mainly mothers—talking aloud to one another about which prestigious school was interested in their child or how their child was learning to ski or play tennis. I was worried about when or whether my four-year-old son was going to walk.

As the spring progressed, so did Seth. He was learning to stand: he stood behind his stroller and used it for balance testing himself by letting go for a few seconds and exploring the feeling of no support. My classes with Carola and in the Feldenkrais training continued. I was not interested in becoming a Feldenkrais practitioner but I wanted to know more about methods that could help both Seth and me. It is fortunate that I was gaining confidence in myself, because soon thereafter Anat decided to quit New York and move her practice to the West Coast.

We were devastated. There had been real hope that Seth would be walking independently soon, and summer was almost upon us. The next day I contacted Charles and arranged for Seth to begin working with him in September. In the meantime with the intention of increasing my knowledge I was embarking on another leg of the Feldenkrais Training. Seth was dependent on what I knew and was learning. I had a shaky faith in my ability to influence Seth's progress. I put all I had learned and everything I intuited, I put my whole heart into working with Seth on my own for July and August. In September I learned that Jay and I would be welcoming a second child: I was pregnant.

In the months leading up to my due date, I let my professional life absorb me and made one more stab at independent producing. I felt pressure to accomplish something concrete in my life outside of Seth and the family before our new baby was born. I worked hard setting up my projects in Hollywood. Even then, however, I sensed that my life was taking a different direction. I continued my evening classes with Carola and kept up my studies in the Feldenkrais training when I was home in New York. It became clear that I was going to have to prioritize what to do about my time outside of the family.

Despite this craziness, I felt calm about having another child. Everything I learned about cerebral palsy helped me understand that Seth's circumstances were not a result of a preexisting condition or a problem with my pregnancy: it was an injury to his brain at birth. However, the experience of Seth's delivery put me on alert. This time I knew what I wanted from a doctor: I wanted a woman who would take into account my prior experience and be empathic.

My pregnancy was smooth and Seth was making incremental progress; he was standing for a few seconds independently, only a few seconds. He was still holding on to the back of his stroller to walk. I was nervous because, thinking of practical matters, I was worried that we were going to need a double stroller. When our daughter, Haya, was born, I kept telling myself, "Be confident. Seth will walk independently one day."

Seth started walking by the time he was four-and-a-half years old (at first on his knees). We enrolled him in a school that normalized our situation to some degree. By five he was walking more, but his speech was still hard to understand. He had aged out of his preschool, and he had two good years of preschool surrounded by children who seemed not so different than he was.

By six years old Seth was fully ambulatory, but first grade was a disaster. Unsympathetic teachers, lots of stairs, and other factors contributed to a year of hell for him (and us). Seth struggled; teachers reported discipline problems and this upset me. Seth was miserable and so were we. We met with the school and realized we had to seek special education for Seth. What a shock! Seth was obviously intelligent but his motor issues inhibited his learning and frustrated him.

Our new focus involved becoming educated about special education. New titles were added to my growing library of special-needs literature. We went through all the machinations of evaluations and applications with our Board of Education. It was very confusing for us and frustrating for Seth. When academics pass a child by, there are discipline problems; we were having them with Seth. He was lagging well behind. He was upset and I was a wreck.

After much work on our part to overcome this stormy time in our voyage, we were relieved and happy when Seth was accepted and began "second grade" at a school for gifted children with special needs. The Stephen Gaynor School felt like a safe haven after all the anxiety of the prior months of testing and school visits and rejections. After a period of adjustment, Seth thrived at Stephen Gaynor. So did we.

Over time I saw my relationship to the orthodox medical world unraveling. We still visited our pediatrician, but I could not imagine discussing with her my breathing work with Carola and the Feldenkrais work I was doing with Seth. I took a further step away from the establishment when I started to visit Dr. Domenick Masiello, a cranial osteopath and homeopath.

Initially I went to Dr. Masiello on a lark (a friend's recommendation) because I was fighting a persistent finger infection and getting no solutions. The initial interview with Dr. Masiello lasted more than two hours. Did I like cold? Hot? What were my sleep patterns? Was I thirsty at night? We discussed Seth and my pregnancy and delivery, my athletic injuries, my relationships. I felt valued.

After a few appointments, the doctor suggested that I step into the adjacent room for an osteopathic treatment. I put up some resistance because I had sought him out for a finger infection in his capacity as a homeopath, but he had gained my trust, so I followed his suggestion, lying down on the treatment table—a table exactly like the countless others I knew from previous physical therapy sessions: from Seth's days with Anat, from his sessions with Susan and Charles. The doctor stood behind me and placed his hands on my head. Less than a minute later out I went. How long I "slept" I cannot say for sure. When I awoke I enjoyed an absolutely unique sense of well-being and openness. There was a lightness and ease I had not felt in months. The feeling lasted into the next day and for a few days afterward.

When I woke up after that first cranial osteopathic session, I asked Dr. Masiello about treating Seth (whom he had never met). He told me there was only one place to go: Dr. Viola Frymann's Osteopathic Center for Children in California. I plunged. Six months later we were on our way to see her. Seth's had progressed only so far with the Feldenkrais work, and treatments with Dr. Frymann were the next logical step.

Dr. Frymann recommended a regular treatment plan for Seth including three one month sessions with her every year; she wanted him tested at the Spitz Clinic in Philadelphia to determine the extent of the insult to his brain. This was the first time we had any specific neurological tests administered. Dr. Frymann introduced us to Peter Springall, a sensory motor learning specialist, who began treating Seth whenever we were having sessions with Dr. Frymann. At Dr. Springall's suggestion we purchased equipment like he had in his office. This enabled us to rigorously follow a home program he recommended where once again I was at the helm of the ship.

There was another development at this time. Yoga had been part of my life since my 20's when I started taking basic hatha yoga classes. After a few years one of my instructors came back from training with B.K.S. Iyengar in India and she introduced this intensive and revolutionary practice to us. I took the opportunity to seek out the Iyengar Institute near Dr. Frymann's office, began classes, and met my first teachers. Soon I was taking class every day and taking workshops, going on retreats. Iyengar teachers were staying with us when they visited New York to teach workshops and Intensives. They worked with Seth and gave us feedback. By that point I had established a pattern: discover what worked for me, and then introduce it to Seth.

Feldenkrais, craniosacral osteopathy, Iyengar: people disputed our non-traditional choices and faulted me for not enrolling Seth in more strenuous mainstream programs of physical and occupational therapy. What I learned is that I had to find what worked for Seth and for the family. I sought out constructive and experienced input and I worked to shut out the naysayers. My task was finding a fine balance between being headstrong and being hard headed.

In today's world people are more open. Brain science shows that what were once "far out" and "alternative" methods of therapy are acceptable or at the very least are considered "complementary" therapies. Add to that today's technology advancements and the result is the elimination of many barriers that existed when Seth was first diagnosed. The landscapes have changed and then nothing has changed. I was, am, and will be the parent of a spectacular special-needs child and his wonderfully unique sister.

Chapter 1

LOGGING
Using a journal to track and guide your journey.

A record kept on a regular basis aboard ship is called a log. The term comes from the fact that these records were originally kept by inscribing information onto shingles cut from logs and hinged so they opened like books.

Fortunately for me, a friend described a journal she kept during a serious illness. She told me how she benefited by keeping notes about what doctors said during her various appointments and how she monitored her progress. I knew I had to do the same. Memory is critical; it is significant and it has consequences. Safeguard it by writing what you can down.

Journaling is a healthy habit to cultivate and has surprising benefits that last forever. I wrote everything down in a journal and it was pivotal to my experience as a mother of a child with special needs. To be sure, it is a helpful practice to have generally. Eventually I maintained a journal about our daughter, Haya, chronicling her medical visits and school conferences as I did Seth's. I recorded random thoughts and observations about both children that included all their illnesses and many of their moods.

As you make your way through this guidebook, use a journal

to chronicle what you learn about yourself as well as what you discover as you explore solutions for your child and family.

Find or buy a notebook you can use for a journal.

A simple notebook will do, nothing elaborate or costly.

I like writing on lined paper and prefer soft, lightweight covers making it easy to roll up and slip into my handbag. One mother I know likes sketch paper, big blank pages, bound in a hardcover. She has big handwriting and drawing talent, whereas I cannot draw a straight line thus needing lines to write on!

Always have a notebook and pen with you. In your busy day carve out a small time—on the same day of the appointment—for a journal entry.

Journal entries can be brief! Be sure to include the important details and then expand if you have time.

I always date my entries and say where I am. Example: November 2, 20__, NY, dining room following Dr. L's appointment.

It is important to date the entries to create a timeline. I like titles for the entry like "A Good Day" and write one line or two. Examples are: "Nancy had no tantrums today," or "Kevin did not take his medicine easily and was difficult at lunch but went to bed easily."

Some of my entries are very short: "Dr. F____'s appointment was this afternoon. Nothing new. Seth was friendly with her." Or, "therapy with Susan went well." (Either could be the entire entry.) "Jane Smith called today. She wants me to meet so and so..." (another parent? therapist?) This makes the name and number easy to retrieve. Names of books I heard about and contacts are in one place. Other entries ramble on for a while dealing with frustrations and feelings—depending on how much time I had—but the appointments and consultations are there.

In your entries about doctor visits, write down how you and your child each feel about the practitioner and definitely include what is being prescribed as a course of treatment.

Our impressions of a practitioner are equally important as the recommendations.

For example, in addition to the medical terms or the other words you hear, you can note an appointment like the following:

- "Dr. X was warm and welcoming. S. felt right at home. Am not sure why he is recommending this therapy (write down what it is) but we will try it."

- "Dr. Y 's head nurse wants us to call her next week. Visits with the doctor are rushed but results are positive. Worth staying with her?"

- " I told F's teacher about what we are doing at home.

She suggested to read his homework assignments out loud."

- "Dr. Z did not touch R or look me in the eye and R was miserable, but the doctor did mention the new gene tests."

Give yourself a reasonable timeline for checking back about effectiveness of treatments/strategy balanced with how you feel about the practitioner personally.

Journaling is how we capture the technical and emotional details that are so meaningful for future decisions and for reminders of what has come before.

Seth worked one summer with Stoney, a college baseball player. They spent every morning in a program of monkey bars, trampoline, and stretching based on directions from Dr. Springall. (They also drove around in Stoney's car listening to rock 'n roll!)

As part of the j0b description I asked Stoney to keep a journal of his time with Seth, to report on their activities. The journal starts out describing things like "Seth started on the trampoline. He worked really hard." or "...we wrestled and did some crawling exercises." As the journal progressed, Stoney included notes on how he encouraged Seth, and even snippets of their conversations. The journal became increasingly detailed to include both Seth's reactions and Stoney's emotions about it. The journal attached *a dimension* to the "job." It made for *reflection*. Recently I read over the last entry in Stoney's diary from that summer.

Dear Laura and Jay,

I really appreciate all you have done for me. You made my summer worthwhile. I hope that the time I spent with Seth helped. I wish the best for him to succeed in all that he does. I know he will. It makes me feel good to see the expressions on your faces when Seth accomplishes something. The joy I see in you makes me feel like I have accomplished something too. Seth has really taught me a lot about myself, and life in general. He is a great kid. The experiences and moments we shared will last forever.

"Dear Diary…" has always been part of my life. It took on a different dimension and hue once Seth was diagnosed. Making it a habit as a parent of a child with special needs is an offer you can't refuse.

What we write speaks volumes about who we are and our states of mind. Our words can also impact how we perceive the world and how we will feel going forward.

—Brett Steenbarger writing in *Forbes*

SUGGESTED READING:

Brett Steenbarger's full article "Two Powerful Reasons to Keep a Journal" is available online. As of this printing (January 2017, it can be found at the following address: www.forbes.com/sites/brettsteenbarger/2015/07/10/two-powerful-reasons-to-keep-a-journal/ #2f038f6d4

There are very helpful videos about journaling. I like the following one in particular: "How to Bullet Journal" on YouTube.

Chapter 2

HOME PORT

Becoming aware of your personal style.

"It is not in the stars to hold our destiny but in ourselves."
—William Shakespeare

How you came to being a parent of a special-needs child is not something I can know from where I sit. I imagine it is not something you planned for.

While there is no way to ask *where* you are on your voyage, I suggest stopping for a moment to ask yourself an essential question: "*Who* am I on this journey?"

It is natural to focus on our child. With all our worry and concern it is what we do for our children, all of them. Because we are so caught up in the here and now and with the very real and pressing needs of our family it is helpful to step back, take a breath and assess who we are. It influences how we best deal with what is needed.

Asking certain questions about who we are—passive? assertive? shy? take charge? organized/disorganized?—is how we develop awareness of our personality type and how we deal with challenge and conflict; how we deal with other people. This is what dictates the route we take. We change in many ways during our life, take different and divergent paths. Awareness of who we are as an individual is our home port, our starting point.

Perform a "personal inventory" to identify the strengths and challenges of your personality.

Assessing our personality is different than judging or changing it.

Knowledge of who we are, what situations provide comfort or discomfort, and how we deal with others—especially those in authority—provision us for our voyage with a supply of insight and style. This can be as detailed as undertaking a personality evaluation through Myers-Briggs, or simply considering whether we deal best with *people, things,* or *information.* In the Suggested Reading for this chapter there are diverse resources to help accomplish this task.

There is so much awe, so much magic about doctors—including celebrity doctors like Dr. Oz—which is why we expect so much of them. It is natural to look for an outside authority to be in charge. Initially my attitude towards doctors included both reverence and resentment. Now I see how passive I was during my pregnancy and Seth's delivery. The doctor was matter of fact; he was unconcerned, and so sure of himself that while I was uncomfortable with him it never occurred to me to mistrust him or that he might not know everything. Generally, that was my attitude toward doctors until I recognized that I was being passive. It was not easy at first, but I changed; I took a more active role and started asking questions that I needed to help Seth.

If I knew more, I could have asked for a stress test during the two weeks after Seth's due date; queried whether the days of contractions before my delivery was a sign of prodromal labor, but since this was my first pregnancy I did not know and I relied on the expert—in this case my doctor. During my difficult labor and delivery, I did not have the courage or information to question him or the situation.

How do you react to authority? What are the positives about your style? What are the negatives?

Try not to judge yourself. Learn from the positive and negative experiences rather than having regret.

After Seth's difficult birth not one doctor mentioned—they never said a word—that there was any reason to be concerned about the future. It was me, relying on instinct, who knew something was not right and insisted on a diagnosis. Because it was about my child I went from passive to active overnight. It was impossible to rest until I had the answers that I wanted. I had to be an activist.

I was undeterred in my mission to get everything I could for my son; that is who I became. It took time to get used to my "new self," more assertive and less aggressive, more of a questioning person. I grew secure enough to pursue new avenues of information about what I did not know and to ask questions without rancor. I found out how difficult it is to go into unchartered waters even when our "safe harbor" is not so safe anymore.

It was a process of letting go, followed by latching on, and ultimately steering the vessel myself. In the beginning I came into the doctor-patient relationship believing the doctor had all the answers and it was a gradual evolution to balance what I learned from them and from others with what I trusted inside.

For instance, I genuinely liked and trusted my pediatrician. However, she failed to recognize there was something amiss—even though she had the birth history long before anyone else. At first I listened to her rather than myself—partly because it was my hope that she was right and there was nothing wrong with Seth. I wanted to believe her reassurances: "Wait until he's a year old." "Children develop differently." But I knew. I knew deep down something was wrong. From that point onward, I took hold of the captain's wheel and did not let go.

Take what you learned about yourself from the exercises above and apply it to the job description you have as a parent. Get what you need to do that job by asking questions, writing down the answers and figuring out how to use them to implement solutions.

This is how we "grow up!" It may be difficult giving voice to doubts and fears, but when we delineate those fears, we grow. We must be convinced of our self-worth and learn the "courage" to ask important questions.

Beyond getting the initial information, eventually I worked up the strength I needed to break away from the mainstream. When I did, I saw our pediatrician was capable and familiar, but not particularly supportive of my efforts to pursue alternative solutions. I didn't have anyone else and had to get what I needed from her while sticking to my gut about what I believed was going to help Seth—no matter what she or anyone else said. These were some of my first lessons in balance and politics.

Being headstrong—my personality—supported my efforts to get that help for Seth; to deny the naysayers when we introduced non-conforming therapies. However, sometimes it prevented me from receiving information and support as in the case of the social worker at the hospital or from the massage therapist. I learned the important distinction between being headstrong versus being hard-headed—the latter is rarely a good thing. Willfulness can help with advocacy or it can be a detriment. We need to be aware of how it is working in each situation and find balance.

We are impacted by stress and trauma—of course to different degrees. When we learn from past victories and from past failures we shape our destiny as well as being shaped by such challenges. It depends on the way we embrace—or resist—our trials. Resilience and steadfastness are essential attributes that rely on self-awareness. Having purpose, finding meaning. Knowing more about ourselves makes us better parents for our child—any child—and a better captain of our ship!

SUGGESTED READING:

Many people think of Myers-Briggs when they consider personality types. The following book is especially good: *Gifts Differing: Understanding Personality Type.*

Another valuable book and methodology by Keirsey & Bates is *Please Understand Me: Character and Temperament Types.*

A respected perspective on finding your type comes from Renee Baron in her book, *What Type Am I?: Discover Who You Really Are.*

Chapter 3

SEMAPHORE

Shaping and sending the message
of your child's situation.

"Not only must the message be correctly delivered,
but the messenger himself must be such as to
recommend it to acceptance."
—Joseph Barber Lightfoot

Semaphore is a system of sending messages by holding the arms or
two flags or poles in certain positions according to an alphabetical
code (think railroad signals). Someone witnessing it for the first
time may think semaphore is merely waving poles or flags, yet once
we learn this particular language, we can *read* the reports being sent.

We begin receiving messages from our child's semaphore—
from the moment he is born. His cries, his sleep, every blink of an
eye is his alphabet. What parent does not remember the moment
of recognition when our baby first smiles at us? What a message!

As life goes on we get signals from our child that are more
complicated than smiles and cries and we learn to read them. We
get messages from doctors and teachers, other parents, and from
observing our child when he is interacting with others. Each interaction—medical, social, familial—has its own vocabulary and dialect.

Until our child has language, we communicate for him—interpreting and then conveying his message to others. (This is true of course for a child *without* special needs too.) In the case of our special-needs child we discover when and how to begin telling the outside world about him and about our family's unique situation. His disability may not reveal itself to outsiders at once or it may be so obvious that an explanation is immediately necessary. It depends on our individual situation.

We continually exchange messages—overtly and otherwise—and communicate in multiple dimensions: with words and actions and with body language. We communicate internally—within the family—in one dimension; with different nuances in our communications to and interactions with the external world. Our child watches us and understands and absorbs our messages, many unspoken.

Do a "body check" to determine what messages your stance is sending. Are your shoulders hunched? Is your jaw clenched? What is the tone and loudness of your voice?

We communicate with our whole selves—not only with words but with body language, tone, volume, with whispers or hushed voices, lowered eyes.

Early communications with various therapists and doctors were fraught with emotions and anxieties. I was afraid the therapist would tell me something negative or that I was communicating my anxiety. It was only with experience—including missteps—that I learned to deal with each individual involved in Seth's rehabilitation and education as just that: individuals. I had to sort them out on the spectrum of personalities and foibles, their various positions in the scheme of things.

I developed hyper awareness of how each therapist or doctor or teacher or school administrator affected me, what messages I was sending and what signals they were picking up on. I learned to clamp down on my impulses to respond and react. It took effort to find the balance between what I hoped to hear and what I did hear. So much depended on the messenger.

I grew to understand the part I played in these interactions and how much depended on what I told the practitioner; it depended on my projections as well. Jay helped me with this by role playing or rehearsing with me about what I wanted to say when we were trying new things and making changes or trying to get something across about what I needed. When Seth began to have input the equation changed, although I always had to monitor myself and make space to observe how Seth interpreted the messages and how they impacted him. I was modeling for him. When I sought answers and needed to be assertive, I was careful not to come off as badgering, but also I did not allow people to see me as too easy going when I had to get my point across.

Practice encounters with someone else or in a mirror to get feedback on the messages you are sending.

Working in the mirror helps us see the unspoken messages we send with body language, tone, and volume. Revisit the "body check" at the beginning of this chapter.

When our child has a special need, we gradually become adept at communicating his needs and situation to the greater world. *Gradually* is the operative word because becoming efficient at this takes practice; we go carefully and thoughtfully—carefully and with thought because our dispatches possibly convey stereotypical messages and possible misinformation. Remember a listener has a personal "context" or expectation about what a certain label means.

Sometimes we receive mixed messages regarding our child's situation! How do we convey a message to others when we have yet to decipher it for ourselves? For instance, when we first learned that Seth had cerebral palsy, we received one diagnosis from Dr. C and another more pessimistic diagnosis from a doctor in Boston in a second opinion. That was confusing and scary. In addition to dealing with the news, we had decisions to make about *how* much we shared with the outside world, *how* to do so, and *when*.

Making decisions about when to share what Jay and I were learning or what we thought we knew was illustrated by the time my father came with us for the second opinion. As the doctor delivered his rather pessimistic opinion, I saw my father's crest-fallen face and it was a clear message to me: from that point on I would be the link to and the filter through which any and all information about Seth was transmitted to *everyone*!

Ask yourself what you know and how much you want others to know. Use your journal to write down your current understanding of the situation.

The key here is our current understanding. Give yourself permission not to have all the answers right away; writing down what we know keeps our focus on the present.

Our messages change depending on the audience. I certainly shared differently with close and trusted friends than with extended family or even some close family. It depended on the various people and who they were in my life. The messages and labels were also tailored for those who needed to better understand our situation so they might do the most to help Seth. If our child does not exhibit "differences," it is not always necessary to provide an elaborate description for each person we meet. The level of information shared needs to match our relationship and the situation.

One reason my family was aware that Seth was lagging behind in certain milestones was that I had a niece Seth's age pulling herself to stand before Seth was even sitting up alone. The questions kept coming. We had to give explanations. I hesitated because I knew the labels connoted what may or may not come true. *Disability* covers as much of a spectrum as *autism* or *developmental delays* or *cerebral palsy*.

For example, autism is a collection of behaviors rather than a known biological entity; it is a syndrome rather than an illness. It encompasses a highly variable group of symptoms and behaviors, and there is no way to measure it except by its external manifestations. To someone not aware of these nuances, hearing that a child is autistic may bring assumptions of a particular manifestation— probably based on their own social experiences or impressions. Our challenge and responsibility is deciding when to explain and what to explain and to whom.

Examine what words you use to convey information about your child. How do you tell others about your family's situation without skewing the reality and without imposing stereotypes on others' thinking?

Expressing what our child is able to do or what challenges he has helps others separate who our child is from his condition. Before speaking the label of his diagnosis or a description of his symptoms try describing his unique positive qualities, like the way he smiles or his passion for trucks.

How do we get the insight and the support we need to sort out the messages—often mixed—and discover ways to relay them? The experience of other parents is one way, and those experiences are sometimes on websites or Facebook pages or through personal introductions. Keep in mind that suggestions from other parents are not always appropriate for us and our circumstances.

Enlist the help of a doctor, trusted friend, family member, or therapist to help sort out the message you want to send.

Those who know us best can help give context to the message we hope to convey.

Pivotal is the moment our child begins to speak for himself. This circumstance is well illustrated by an incident at a summer picnic. We were happily sharing our picnic dinner with a family we had gotten to know. Their daughter, Anna, asked her mother why Seth talked like he did, why he was difficult to understand.

I answered her immediately. "Everyone has challenges, Anna,"

I began. I was going on to say, "Seth has some differences that make it hard for him to do things you and Haya and I do easily and talking is one of them."

Seth put his hand on my arm to stop me. He turned to Anna and said—as clearly as he ever spoke anything—"I have a friend in California. He listens to me in the noisiest room. He understands everything I say. When he isn't sure, he asks me to say it again."

That was the last time I needed to answer for Seth. He answered Anna for himself, putting some of the responsibility on her to understand him.

Stop yourself from speaking for your child in every situation. Let your child use his voice when he indicates he is ready.

Giving our child room to test the waters and make mistakes is a way to be supportive.

It did not take long for Seth to know that he is not like others. There were unkind and judgmental glances, overt and implied ridicule. We learned a lexicon of responses to questions that were put to us and eventually to Seth. We had to evolve over many stages to answer appropriately in all the situations that arose. It took discussion and practice and it meant paying close attention and exercise discipline.

At each developmental stage, each medical visit, each social or educational interaction, Jay and I acquired new vocabulary, expanding the lexicon to communicate with and for our son;

developing the semaphore to stay on track. We grew to understand what Seth was communicating to us, how to communicate for him, and how to help him find his own voice to communicate for himself.

SUGGESTED READING:

ChangingMinds.org provides a helpful and informative list of different messages and emotions expressed through body language.

Chapter 4

MAPPING

Defining yourself as the parent
of a special-needs child.

*"There are times as a parent when you realize that
your job is not to be the parent you always imagined
you'd be, the parent you always wished you had.
Your job is to be the parent your child needs, given
the particulars of his or her own life and nature."*
—Ayelet Waldman

Parents go through developmental stages just as children do, and it
is healthy to be forgiving, to appreciate hindsight, and to change.

We are first-time parents or maybe second-time parents but
*we become a different parent when our child is diagnosed with a
special need.*

When Seth was first diagnosed, I became the parent of
a "patient." My questions relied on answers from the mainstream—the *allopathic*—medical community, the community
of conventional means of treatment. It is what I knew. I called
our pediatrician, Dr. L. I called pediatric physical therapists like
Amy and Susan. Because Seth was a first child and I was a new
parent, I was limited by the conventional medical model; I had

no basis for comparison. Over time my world enlarged. I went into relatively uncharted waters because my back pain demanded it. By following this less-traveled route, I uncovered methods that impacted me and that eventually made a big difference for Seth. I found myself drawn in an alternative direction that today is called *integrated* or *complementary* medicine.

Simultaneously I became a different kind of parent because I grew as a person.

Who are you as a "patient?" Think about how it is different from who are you as the parent of a "patient."

You may discover that you are more assertive on behalf of your child than you ever were for yourself.

I stopped being passive, which began in earnest when I stopped being intimidated by the "experts." I needed experts for sure, but I had to become more informed myself to ask better questions—questions that would lead to real solutions for Seth.

My relationship to medical professionals changed. I began to see more clearly what I had to do to engage with the establishment in order to get answers. I found that many in the medical community saw a diagnosis—just using the word "patient" seemed to make it so!—so I always tried to have them see Seth as Seth. The osteopaths like Frymann and doctors like Kessler, therapists like Anat saw an integrated totality and emphasized the importance of looking at the whole patient. I learned from them.

We were always getting input and instructions and getting directives to mimic therapy for Seth—positions to avoid and ways of handling him, strategies to help him—but what I mostly wanted was to indulge in motherhood and babyhood. Not everything had to be about "making things better" for him, when what could be better than cuddling and loving and playing?

Establish a schedule for working with your child on their therapies if it is appropriate. At the end of this work time, be free to separate the "captain" self from the "mom" self.

We do not want our child to feel that when we are together it is always "work."

Another example of the way Jay and I grew as parents was that we began to recognize that our child as an individual. During much of Seth's early life, it felt like he was an extension of me. As any parent would, I made all of the decisions about eating, sleeping, playing. Now decisions about his care took on new meaning. I had to view him as an individual and determine how each decision affected him medically, physically, mentally, *holistically*. And I had to be sensitive to how I researched and determined each decision because the way I carried out those responsibilities impacted him too.

Whenever we went for a consultation or appointment nurses and doctors asked Jay and me zillions of questions about my pregnancy and delivery, questions about Seth's developmental lags. I had to rehash the painful events around Seth's birth or describe and all his developmental lags: no, he was not pulling himself to stand; and, yes, he drooled a lot or no, he did not crawl. In the beginning Seth was almost always nearby or in earshot when we talked to the doctors or when we were discussing things with the therapists and other professionals.

Seth was not just a little person whose treatment was being determined, he was a young child overhearing a discussion about him. Even at a young age children comprehend attitude, emotion, and concern for them. Intuitively I felt Seth could be influenced by his perceptions of these adult conversations. I just knew he might be influenced by what he "heard" and "saw"—what my *semaphore* was telling him. (See the *Semaphore* chapter for more information about messaging.)

Dr. Frymann and Dr. Springall, Feldenkrais, Iyengar, and Dr. Milton Erickson stressed the importance of leaving the future wide open, of removing obstacles, especially by not listening—or letting our child listen—to typical prognoses. It was Dr. Frymann who put an end to Seth (and Haya) being in earshot of adult conversations.

These doctors and thinkers said that *providing a child with the opportunities to evolve is the most important job of parents.* One good way to avoid setting limits is to keep children away from hearing discussions of their circumstances or from hearing the process of decisions regarding them. Adult conversations must be kept between adults at all stages and settings.

If we discuss the possibility that our child may or may not learn to do something within his earshot, he may doubt his ability and the prophecy can be self-fulfilling. Send the right signals! "Interpretation follows the mouth," is a well-known Talmudic saying. Beginning in infancy children rely on responses from their parents to help them make sense of the world. Very young children receive impressions of adult conversations from tone and body language because they have no other language, but these are messages nonetheless.

The next time you are having an adult conversation with a doctor, friend or spouse, be aware of your child's presence, what they are hearing in words and tone, body language and from the other messages you are sending—spoken and unspoken.

Providing our child with information not deliberately meant for him can influence his self-perception.

When to let a child in on decisions or on more information constantly evolves. As he grows, we can calibrate our conversations and make decisions about when and how much to include him.

Dr. Frymann was always enlightening me about being a better parent. In listening to and absorbing her teachings, I began thinking more and more of our family as a mobile. When one piece of a mobile moves, other pieces are affected and have to move to regain balance. If one piece is too heavy, the mobile shifts and loses the balance. Because she saw her patients in the context of a whole family and wanted her patients to have self-awareness, discipline, and limits, I learned to think like that too, and I always came back to the concept of the mobile.

The doctor pointed out Seth's rivalry with his sister and his anger about not having me all to himself. I reacted by thinking that it would be typical for siblings to compete for attention. Initially I chalked it up to being the mother; later I looked at how I contributed to their stress and vowed to be less apprehensive about Seth's future.

Most people tend to be hard on themselves. I certainly have a harsh inner critic. It was interesting to see that as I dealt more positively with my anxiety and my feelings of inadequacy, the darker disagreements faded between my children and we all moved around more freely!

Researchers support what Dr. Frymann stressed: they say that the most important environmental factor in children's early lives is the way their parents interact with them. When a parent's reactions are sensitive and measured, children are more likely to learn that they have the capacity to cope with feelings even when intense and unpleasant. I encourage you to explore this concept by reading Paul Tough's writings on how children succeed.

Examine your reactions. Are they sensitive and measured? Is your mobile balanced? Moving freely? What part of the mobile are you? What can you do to stabilize and balance the other elements?

One secret to good mothering is being a well-contented mother. Addressing our own needs helps us provide a steadying influence.

Naturally, I was a different parent to Haya after being a parent to Seth—like all parents who must find new ways to parent each child and in each of his developmental stages. We are a different parent for each child and it is different for them and for us at each level of their development (and ours).

As Dr. Alison Gopnik writes in *The Carpenter and the Gardener*, the joy of being a parent is about loving our child...

...from the moment-by-moment physical and psychological joy of being with this particular child, and in that child's moment-by-moment joy in being with you. Love doesn't have goals or benchmarks or blueprints, but it does have a purpose. Love's purpose is not to shape our beloved's destiny but to help them shape their own. In fact, the very point of commitment, nurture and culture is to allow variation, risk and innovation. Even if we could precisely shape our children into particular adults, that would defeat the whole evolutionary purpose of childhood.

As parents we go forward and are captains of our ship when we are equipped with self-knowledge, the fulcrum of our family mobile. Skills acquired through insight into our personal style and our self-education provide us the maps needed to leave the harbor and go out into the world as effective navigators for our child and our family.

SUGGESTED READING

Dr. Gopnik's book *The Gardener and the Carpenter: What the New Science of Child Development Tells Us about the Relationship between Parents and Children* is informative and very easy to read. It is impacting current thinking.

Train Go Sorry: Inside a Deaf World by Leah Hager Cohen is a favorite book because it reads like a novel. It provides another perspective on being parents in the world of special needs as it is told from the perspective of a child whose parents have special needs.

Chapter 5

RAISING ANCHOR
Exploring your approach to research and advocacy on behalf of your child.

"Wherever you go, go with all your heart."
—Confucius

Parents of a child with special needs have relationships with doctors and other professionals and caregivers that exceed the relationships of most parents. Our relationships with the people who diagnose and treat our child are very complex. We need them. We desperately hope that they will succeed. Maybe we believe that if they like us—the parents—they will help our child more.

We want miracles, magic. And these professionals hold the promise of those miracles. We often make them into gods. Maintain the professionalism of the relationship and demand the most from them rather than working to be their favorite patient/parent.

What is a "special need?" Who is a "special-needs child?"

Many children receive their diagnosis under an "umbrella" such as autism or cerebral palsy, but the special needs of each individual range in degree throughout the aspects of their physical, mental, and social well-being. Some conditions may be more manageable than others, but all require some level of accommodation, usually arranged for or carried out by us.

When a child is diagnosed with a special need, it is traumatic and confusing for everyone. There is shock and heartbreak. It is difficult enough to attain an even keel emotionally, never mind get information at such a critical time. Our worlds are shattered.

It is tough to know what to believe or feel about anything— the orthodox medical establishment or the un-orthodox medical establishment; what one expert says and what another expert says. Then there is the chatter on the Internet (which can be helpful but also confusing.)

And the labels! They set us down a path with many branches. Some branches bear fruit; others are dangerous and remember: not one size fits all. It is important that we grasp as much information as we can (even when we are in shock); it is important to feel comfortable to ask questions and to express ourselves. How do we interpret a prognosis and handle our expectations and everyone else's? It can be a nightmare of tears, fears, and isolation.

How full an understanding—beyond the labels—do you have of the facets of your child's disability? Examine the sources of your information.

To dispel the expectations that come with a label, it is important to understand how our child's particular special need affects him personally. Then we can decide how to convey this information to others.

We are the first and earliest messengers for our child in the world and it is important to be careful about using labels that mean different things to different people whether we are seeking information or explaining ourselves.

Remember to keep in mind that many people have preconceived notions of labels like *cerebral palsy, autism, developmental delay,* or *dyslexia,* and it becomes our job to define these labels depending on the particular circumstance.

Soon I was planning my approach to parents and friends, which meant being very thoughtful and aware. It was necessary for me to be the arbiter/interpreter and to help them with their anxiety and bewilderment. Perhaps I was in denial, but I found it hard to imagine Seth as anything other than perfect, never mind possibly impaired, ill, or in danger. I had to put the best spin on things for myself as well as everyone else.

The attitude we adopt for everyone else's benefit to reassure them that we are doing everything possible to insure our child's future is the message that counts when dealing with doctors, nurses, therapists, parents, friends and family.

Consider how your attitude to the outside world affects your inner world.

It is important to be positive but it is just as important to be realistic.

Everyone has their own style when dealing with challenges (as we discussed in the *Home Port* chapter). Mine was to discover all I could to establish a course and embrace it wholeheartedly. I developed relationships with the caregivers, doctors, therapists, whoever was involved with us. I kept notes. I was organized. As

Admiral David Jeremiah said, *"You can't roll up your sleeves if you're wringing your hands."*

Make a list of both the personal qualities and professional opinions of doctors and other professionals involved with your child. Separate the two to be sure you are pursuing options that best benefit your child.

We cannot allow our desire to be liked by the people treating our child to limit our scrutiny or the rigor we expect of them.

It is important to examine and reexamine the level that we rely on experts. It is easy to lose perspective of the big picture and be swayed by daily progress and challenges. One way to maintain equilibrium is to use our journal; looking back on it may give us needed perspective (see the chapter on *Logging*).

The concept that there is "something wrong" with our child is difficult to grasp, and then to figure out how to live with it—to say nothing of explaining it to others—is frightening. Many of us may hesitate exploring or probing too deeply at first for fear of what we might find. There is also the problem of who to listen to and who to trust.

Other personal styles, attitudes and fears play a part in our individual experience. For instance, Seth received a diagnosis of cerebral palsy, but I did not contact United Cerebral Palsy right away. Now I realize that I was scared about what I might find there. I wanted to believe Seth's condition was so mild that the early intervention I was orchestrating was going to be enough to ensure his normal development, his normal integration into the world. The thought of something more severe was out of the reach of my imagination and I wanted to keep it that way.

Most of the parents I have met or interviewed say that they responded as I did during some phase of coming to terms with their child's diagnosis of special needs.

If your child has a specific condition that has a central organization dedicated to that condition, contact them for information. Today.

Established organizations can offer detailed information, referrals to caregivers, and support groups. They are a helpful—sometimes essential—first step.

Whether we have an organization to rely on or not, eventually we have to plunge in and get educated. The Internet is a powerful tool, and offers a plethora of sources of information and forums that provide easy access to others' experiences and opinions. Beware of websites that end in ".com" rather than ".org" and keep track of your investment of time in forums. You are looking for information and support and want to avoid "analysis paralysis" or a sales pitch. It is easy to get carried away!

Many individuals I relied on and interacted with influenced how I felt, what I believed, and what I hoped for. My pediatrician gave me praise. Dr. G kept saying all the predictors looked good. Charles said Seth would walk normally and he could not do anything that Susan and others were not doing. The occupational therapist had confidence. I clung to them.

And then I took a few leaps. In our case it was because Seth was stymied. After two and a half years there was little if any progress. Opportunities presented themselves. When we plunged into first the Feldenkrais work with Anat when Seth was not yet three, and three years later when he began to work with Dr. Frymann, we observed major changes. It was Anat and Dr. Frymann who helped Seth fulfill his promise.

Slowly research outside the confines of "established" medical practice if it is appropriate. Gauge your reaction to unfamiliar therapies/information. Test the waters with your comfort level.

The purpose of our research is to uncover what is going to help a child meet his optimal self. We are the best witnesses because we know him the best, and if and when we see a solution that is working, we must pursue it.

I was fortunate I had the advantage of exploring, delving into unusual and out-of-the-ordinary routes. There were financial consequences for us, however. (See the *Storms at Sea* chapter.) Yet we never stopped believing in Seth and what we could do for him because of what I was learning.

I enjoyed the opportunities to explore new methods—Feldenkrais, Carola's work, osteopathy, cranial osteopathy, Iyengar, biofeedback neurotherapy—because my mind was opened to the brain's plasticity and the miracle of the body. Many around me considered these pursuits a bit "kooky." What I knew was that Seth was making progress. There was nothing anyone could say to contradict that.

The challenge for a first-time parent of a child with special needs means paying close, thoughtful attention while trying to stay one step ahead. This is hard work. Our children are diagnosed, but we are not offered much besides the labels. In *Far From the* Tree, Andrew Solomon quotes Jerome Groopman in "The New Yorker:"

> Language is as vital to the physician's art as the stethoscope or the scalpel. Of all the words the doctor uses, the name he gives the illness has the greatest weight. The name of the illness becomes part of the identity of the sufferer.

Sometimes there is too much information. I did not have the option of doing an Internet search when I was raising Seth, but I wonder how well I would have sorted the countless pages of .org, .com, and blinking ads, and found the most effective methods instead of facing "analysis paralysis." This is especially true for diagnoses such as cerebral palsy, developmental disabilities, and autism, where the label applies to a vast array of symptoms, outcomes, and therapies.

There were varying opinions about one thing or another all the time. I tried to focus on Seth in the present moment while also putting in place a methodology that could serve him over the long term.

SUGGESTED READING

Many parents are familiar with the works of T. Berry Brazelton, whose works were a grounding influence for Jay and me. I recommend his book *On Becoming a Family: the Growth of Attachment*, in particular.

In keeping with the message throughout *Uncommon Voyage* that we learn from and support one another, I heartily encourage you to read the stories of others through the Boston Women's Health Book Collective. Their book *Ourselves and Our Children: a Book by and for Parents* is now out of print, but they have many other wonderful titles on their web site, www.ourbodiesourselves.org.

Chapter 6

SHIP'S OFFICERS

**Embracing the joys and challenges in an intimate
relationship as parents of a special-needs child.**

"A friend is one before whom I may think aloud."
—Ralph Waldo Emerson

Jay and I always knew we wanted children. When Seth was born
our focus shifted from us as a couple to us as a family of three. We
were ecstatic and our lives were joyfully consumed with him from
the beginning, and more so—differently—after the diagnosis. We
unconditionally committed ourselves to Seth and the view that all
children are different—all parents are different! No one knows ahead
of time what her child will be like. Yet, I cannot deny the stress we felt
and the worry we had that was ever present and I cannot minimize
the way it permeated our relationship and became part of its fabric.

The stress of raising a child with special needs is a huge element
in a relationship. It makes a partnership vulnerable. We are each
reacting in different ways to the stress of our situation. Some of us
are crushed by a child's diagnosis and others are inspired to tackle
the issues with gusto. There are differences of opinion about care,
the division of labor, and each of us has our individual reaction
to the situation.

Sharing the care of any child with an intimate partner means dividing the load and figuring out how to carry the weight. When a child with special needs is factored in, the pressure increases exponentially. Lack of time and financial considerations are issues; so are social stresses that include relationships with family near and far and people in the wider world. The responsibilities themselves may feel at odds with a romantic ideal.

Examine the health of your relationship. Is the focus you are putting on your child affecting or weakening your marital relationship? Are you embracing your parenting differences and actively listening?

We ask a great deal of ourselves and our partner. The first thing to accept is that neither of us is perfect, and neither is wholly responsible.

The first order of business is the "business" of dividing responsibilities—and determining the balance of responsibility. Some assignments in the care of our child may go to *alloparents*, individual helpers outside of our personal relationship. Work to enlist that help. Recognize how their help is important while remaining different from the help gotten from a partner.

Mothers, fathers, grandmothers and grandfathers, uncles and aunts, siblings, cousins and even friends: these helpers provide us with a unique network of care. They combine to help us take care of our children. We have important relationships with them. The intimate relationship that belongs to a couple stands apart from these. Jay and I saw how important it was to carve out time for ourselves and wrestle with things between us so we at the very least understood each other's viewpoint.

Are each of you using your particular strengths to best benefit your child? Set a minimum initial commitment of one half-hour of uninterrupted time together every day for a "business meeting" to refine these roles and treat that time as sacrosanct: no screens, no talk of kids, no complaining. LISTEN to each other.

Our responsibilities may not be "equal," but we are working towards a common goal. Thirty minutes a day seems like a lot but it is crucial. Seeing ourselves as a team helps to protect our couple relationship.

Jay and I faced our situation from very different vantage points. Two feelings existed in me: I desired to share everything with Jay about what we were doing to help Seth, and at the same time I reined in the impulse to reveal my deepest anxieties and sadness completely. I was unable to "let it all down." I wanted to shield him—and others in the family—from doubts and anxieties that I believed I could deal with better than most people. I believed in being the optimist for the two of us and that I had to buoy everyone else too. The more I did it, the more I became that person.

Jay's energy often focused on converting worry to positive action. He was diligent about safety issues. He figured out logistics and made sure that structures were in place beginning with protection on the school playground and extending to protocols in college that ensured Seth's physical well-being in case of emergency. We all have different strengths, and are of different character and there are variations in knowledge and insight among us. The intersection of these differences lends relationships the opportunity to distribute responsibility while remaining balanced.

As is the case for many parents, my focus shifted from outside our home to inside it when Seth was born, and even more so when he was diagnosed. In particular this affected my work pursuits. After the diagnosis I began spending every spare minute researching and making appointments, interviewing and meeting doctors and therapists, calling people, doing everything I knew how to do. I took up this job enthusiastically and it satisfied my need to be actively doing everything I could.

My commitment to our child and to marriage with Jay overcame any resentment I felt or feel today about giving up work in Hollywood and on Broadway. I surrendered my fantasy of what family and work balance I might have created. New opportunities arose because I did become a stay-at-home mother. In time I surrendered to what life was giving me, giving us—Jay and Seth, Jay and me, Seth and me, and Jay and Seth and me—and adapted myself and my world to the reality of it.

Value yourself and your work as a parent. Be sure your roles and parenting responsibilities feel fair.

Awareness of this shift of responsibility helps partners avoid resentment.

By the time our daughter, Haya, was in school, Jay and I began holding family meetings, and it meant a great deal to our growth as co-parents. In real time we learned together about the children and their relationship—not only to each other but to each of us.

In family meetings conflicts and feelings received ample ventilation. Nuances of the children's interaction were revealed, and I was able to grasp more of their struggles with themselves and with each other, as well as with their father and me and us with them. (I expand on the role of family meetings in the *Shipmates* chapter.) We had the advantage of knowing our children better from these meetings, and this helped when we made decisions about simple plans or deciding more momentous things.

Being parents used up a great deal of our energy as a couple. Jay and I needed energy for the family and we needed a lot of extra energy because of Seth. Time alone became harder and harder to find and we came to the important realization that time for each other was essential—demanded—so that we could continue to rely on one another and value our "couple" relationship. We needed to nurture the part of our relationship that was outside of being parents. We renewed our commitment to restore and support each other because we knew otherwise we had less to give.

It took a lot of arranging but we got away for a long weekend shortly after Haya was born—time for just the two of us. We needed this time to learn that children thrive without parents committing every moment, every thought to them. While we were away and Seth was out of the hovering gaze of his expectant parents, he took his first independent steps walking toward us on his own when we returned.

Seth's developmental leap deeply affected Jay and me. It was a positive occurrence that we shared in equally, each of us experiencing the pride and the hope in Seth's accomplishment. This development shot us through with a sense of hope and reignited our commitment to him and to the family. Two keys to our success were conscious practice and a division of labor.

Release yourself from the responsibility of producing and witnessing every aspect of your child's progress. Rely on alloparents and give your relationship with your partner the attention and respect it warrants.

Accepting that we may not be present or responsible for every progression our child makes means we can share credit and rejoice in the accomplishment rather than in "ownership" of it.

We grew into being parents of a special-needs child because we grew as individuals, as a couple, as partners. We each had to sort out emotions, learning to live in the seat of our individual disappointments while trying to support one another. We came to parenting with the unique experiences of how each of us was raised. Those early lessons informed our first steps; then we determined together how our family would incorporate them.

We tried to focus on the part of ourselves that existed outside of being parents and parents of a child with special needs. As a couple we cycled through individual struggles and couple struggles. We grappled with unanticipated financial demands. We discovered different approaches to being parents. Over time Jay and I learned how important it was to thrash things out between us first, inviting Seth or Haya or both of them to participate afterward in select aspects of decision making. This was something we learned over time and that had to be *practiced* while nurturing and protecting our relationship.

SUGGESTED READING:
The conversations explored by Kathleen Mates-Younman in her *Couples Therapy Workbook: 30 Guided Conversations to Re-Connect Relationships* help us reconnect to our spouses.

Reading *Rick and Bubba's Guide to the Almost Nearly Perfect Marriage* reminds us that "perfect" is not really the goal of marriage!

Chapter 7

TRAVELING COMPANIONS
Determining which individuals and
therapies to take on board.

*"Driven by the conviction that there must be someone
who can cure, we take our children over the surface
of the whole earth, seeking the one who can heal.
We spend all the money we have and we borrow until
there is no one else to lend. We go to doctors good and
bad, to anyone, for only a wisp of hope."*
—Pearl S. Buck

Within a year of diagnosis, my Seth file was bulging with different doctor and therapist reports, while my personal journal was filling with thoughts, observations and desires about Seth and everything that was happening to us. And, yet, when I reflect on Seth's early childhood, instead of just a series of appointments and episodes of hope and despair, I see the progression through and to methods of care that guided his development.

My personal style had an imprint on what happened and who happened. At the same time I never stopped hoping I would find one doctor to give me the answers and an overview, to help me map my voyage. It did not happen. There never was and there never is a one-size-fits-all solution.

As tempting as it may be to "hand over" our child to those providing care and treatment, we must remain stewards of his care and continually evaluate who provides it. The key is to evaluate on an ongoing basis the effectiveness of methods and look as dispassionately as possible at the individuals providing care for our child. This means review and assessment at reasonable intervals. This is also true as we land on the education continuum. (For a further exploration of educational issues, see the chapter titled *Naval Academy*.)

Set an amount of time (two months, six weeks, one year) to keep the "status quo" with established medical practitioners while researching and being open to other options.

Time allows us to evaluate our relationship with a doctor or therapist and determine if it is worth staying with them for their expertise or if they are providing reassurance without progress.

During this time, I had to get used to the fact that I was in charge—whether it was in the direct administration of the doctor/therapists advice or in coordinating the efforts of the people involved and keeping oversight of them. I wrestled with issues of trust, assessing the professionals. Eventually I moved from the allopathic (the established) to osteopathy and Feldenkrais and other "alternative" interventions. It is not for everyone but it worked for me. The recent revolution in brain science puts many of these complementary therapies more into the mainstream. In any event, I found it important to make the distinction between how I felt about individual practitioners as opposed to new and different modalities.

We may like one doctor and not another. Question yourself. Ask: "Why?" Some factors may include whether or not the doctor looks us in the eye and listens. How comfortable do we feel asking questions? How organized is the office? Is the doctor making time for us or just rushing us through? Are we "in love" because the doctor seems to have all the answers?

What feelings do you have about the doctor's bedside manner? How does the practitioner interact with your child? Is it balanced with their suggestions regarding care? Be honest. Voice concerns. Show up for appointments on time and follow directions.

Reviewing notes in a journal helps with the important task of taking responsibility for our part in the doctor/patient relationship. The journals we keep reflect the truth of our perspective over time.

Our relationships to the professional and medical communities are fostered in a relatively narrow and dependent atmosphere. Understandably we do not trust ourselves to question, probe, challenge, and investigate, *at first*.

After paying attention to the doctors and/or therapists treating and working with our child over a reasonable period of time, continue to get to the core of what is going to work for our child by observing him, by doing research (read, talk to others) and exploring some more!

Take comfort in those who offer you the most insight and support and get accustomed to all you are learning to make new discoveries. Make space in your mind for as much as possible without being stupid or carried away on an ocean of blind trust.

Our minds are opened to new possibilities as we gain knowledge and confidence.

In addition to the doctors and therapists we need to closely question individuals who present themselves as healers. Good practitioners in any field never stop studying, taking and offering courses, developing themselves to become more effective, with the constant stimulation of information and exposure.

Research the individuals involved in your child's care to determine their qualifications and training.

Keep in mind that some of the standards regarding "professionals" differ from state to state. It is up to us to question a practitioner, to know his/her qualifications and get answers for what we want to know. Recognize experts and listen to their advice, but remember experts are not always wearing white coats and people in white coats are not always experts.

When we took Seth for an evaluation to Dr. Springall, the sensorimotor developmentalist, we found that he based his work on the findings of Glenn Doman, the founder and head of the Institutes for the Achievement of Human Potential. In his book, *What to Do about Your Brain-Injured Child,* Doman's work emphasizes the brain rather than the body. I felt that Springall functioned in a way that reinforced methods that we were already finding effective for Seth.

As I studied Doman's work I saw how it synchronized with what I was learning about the philosophy of Moshe Feldenkrais, the osteopath Andrew Still, and the works of Dr. William Sutherland. It was all relevant and I was further reassured about the decisions I was making for Seth and for me. These methods took into account the body's inherent therapeutic force that I believed in then and believe in now.

Determine if the professionals around you have an overarching philosophy of care. Are they coordinating within that philosophy to get at "holistic" treatment?

Holistic does not have to mean "new age." It simply means that you and practitioners are looking at the whole child and how each system affects others.

Medical professionals and our community of family and friends were often confused by our choices, questioning techniques they had never heard of. While I am sure most of them were acting out of concern for us, at times it felt as if everyone thought we were crazy.

When I took Seth for a routine pediatric checkup after he was working with Anat for two months, Dr. L. also noted the differences in him. She asked me what we were doing and I told her Feldenkrais work. Her eyes went blank. Another time she referred to it as "witchcraft." After the second or third encounter on this subject—though we continued to see her for routine checkups—I stopped sharing any details with her and referred only to Seth's "therapy."

In the meantime I learned the value of finding allies—people who supported my decisions; who saw why I made the choices I believed were best for Seth. When I did find them, I latched on to them.

Early on the pediatrician's doubts and questioning would have shaken my confidence. Not anymore. Now I had knowledge. My first-hand experience through study and exploration gave me confidence and hope in a course of treatment, and I conveyed that informed optimism to those caring for our child and to our child himself.

Ask questions and request resources so you have everything you need to better comprehend therapies and treatments.

If we are not able to easily articulate to others what a doctor or therapist is doing for and with our child—if we stammer and seem unsure in describing it to others—we may not have a solid understanding of it ourselves.

We wanted to leave "no stone unturned," so we went to a neurologist in New York to consider laser surgery on Seth's spine (he was not a candidate.) Though the doctor's report reflected Seth's achievements, it referred to "Seldencrest [sic] physiotherapy."

Her complete ignorance about Feldenkrais work and her failure to ask questions about it—her inability even to spell the name properly when this philosophy was core to Seth's care—alienated me.

Listen to your developing intuition. Is what is happening with your child in sync with what the doctor is telling you? What do you observe in your child that supports or contradicts your belief in the efficacy of treatments?

Observation must include an awareness of our child's possibly—changing physical attributes as well as his demeanor during and after appointments or treatments.

Dr. G, our highly respected pediatric orthopedist, was positive and seemed to appreciate Seth's personality and humor; I liked him very much. Yet he wanted me to give up Susan and the other therapists and use the therapists in his clinic who were not trained in the NDT (Bobath) method.

The doctor's office was quite a distance from our home and this meant turning Seth's world—and mine—upside down. Frequent visits would have meant an additional level of time commitment that would affect the entire family's schedule.

I stood my ground and did not acquiesce to him because Seth was already reaping the benefits of the Bobath method with our established therapists, and *not doing so worked better for our family.*

Determine the balance between effectiveness of treatment and the basic logistics of getting to and from where it is being offered or especially how your child reacts to the doctor/therapist.

We can trust and like someone, but that does not mean our life revolves around them.

In extreme circumstances as in the situation of a rare disability where there may be only one or two practitioners trained or known to be successful or who come so totally recommended, of course make any kind of accommodation possible. In our case we went to the other side of the country to get what we needed for Seth from Dr. Frymann at considerable sacrifice.

Determine how much stress will result from pursuing a solution that is far from your home or will incur exorbitant expense.

It is not a bad thing to choose comfort and ease as a priority. We are affected by the stress of a situation and that detracts from the effectiveness of a solution.

When there was conflicting information from different professionals, I initially looked to the experts and to our pediatrician for the answer about what to do. Later when Anat came into the picture, I let her—not a doctor or other *experts*—take control of many aspects. At that point I was committed to the Feldenkrais philosophy that Anat was carrying out with Seth and trusted in its benefits for him and I trusted her.

When it came to Dr. Springall who specialized in sensory motor learning, I knew this was the right thing for Seth. I could see it working for him. This specialist was evaluating Seth in multiple respects and writing up a program for him to do at home and it was not dissimilar to Feldenkrais work. I was at ease and confident.

There was no space between what we were doing and how I felt about it. After working with Anat and Dr. Frymann and after an Iyengar practice—Seth looked different. I used to say "his eyes are set different in his head." I felt his energy. It felt like a miracle, something completely non-judgmental. I am not saying he walked, but he was a changed person.

What I observed in Seth after his treatments with Anat and later Dr. Frymann reassured me. I trusted what I saw: Seth was more free, more balanced, at ease, happier, less rigid.

Continue to examine your relationships with all those providing care for your child to determine if the course of treatment is (still) beneficial.

Be comfortable knowing that what works for your child at age three is not necessarily the right solution at age six. We need awareness of our emotional attachments to each person providing care, and we need to continue providing opportunities for our children, even if and when it means moving on.

I worked hard to find people to provide tangible, long-term help for Seth. Once those initial, valuable individuals became involved—people like Susan, Seth's first physical therapist—they provided trustworthy professional help including referrals. Susan, Dr. G, the pediatric podiatrist, were valuable early advisors and interventionists. I took their advice. I took up their referrals. When I encountered other methodologies, I sometimes steered away from them and moved onto others. Often as I took someone new on board, others were asked to disembark.

Good traveling companions are essential, no matter what part of our voyage they share or for how long. They greatly enrich the journey. Take care in choosing them.

SUGGESTED READING:

I have great respect for Dr. Glenn Doman, and found the book *What to Do about Your Brain-Injured Child: or Your Brain-Damaged, Mentally Retarded, Mentally Deficient, Cerebral-Palsied, Epileptic, Autistic, Athetoid, Hyperactive, Attention Deficit Disordered, Developmentally Delayed, Down's Child* to be a tremendous resource.

The practice of yoga became a permanent healing presence in the life of our family. Sonia Sumar's book, *Yoga for the Special Child: a Therapeutic Approach for Infants and Children with Down Syndrome,* Cerebral Palsy, and Learning Disabilities provides a wonderful introduction to yoga's benefits for children with special needs.

Bobbi Clennell is a senior Iyengar yoga teacher and IYAGNY faculty member. Her book, Watch Me Do Yoga, can be found on her website, www.bobbyclennell.com.

Chapter 8

COURSE CORRECTION
Transforming self on both
personal and professional levels.

"To travel is to take a journey into yourself."
—Danny Kaye

Two things happened to me because I ventured out of a safe harbor into the "alternative" world of osteopathy, cranial osteopathy, Feldenkrais, Carola Speads, and Iyengar yoga. First I found ways to help Seth. Whatever methods I tried, how it was named, whether it was mainstream or alternative—it did not matter because I could see that it worked for him.

Secondly, marriage, motherhood, and the opportunities for Seth awakened me and encouraged me to reconsider what was meaningful to me. I believed in the power of the mind, the unique and unparalleled capacity and energy of the brain and the human spirit. Everything I was learning made me more sure of what I knew and I intuited there was more, much more to study and explore. This was exciting!

How "fortunate" that my back pain landed me with a physical therapist, Annie, who was interested in a wide range of methods that were rarely mentioned in those days. She herself was just beginning to dip into these treatments and therapies. They were only starting to be discussed and were outside the mainstream physical therapy world. She was the first to open my mind and raise my awareness about what was "out there."

Annie sketched out a preliminary course, showing me major therapeutic landmarks—the alternatives I had—on the horizon. I began venturing outside the harbor—playing it safe at first and gradually gaining knowledge, experience, and confidence. Once I added details to that map—essentially becoming the cartographer of our voyage—I had sufficient courage to set sail. I gave into being a different person: trusting what I was learning.

Because of Annie's persistence and my willingness—call it curiosity or intuition— I eventually embraced the Feldenkrais method. A pursuit of cranial osteopathy followed logically. At first I listened and I admit I was resistant. After Seth was diagnosed, thankfully, Annie never let up and I started learning and studying. I continued to discover and explore this legitimate world of body/mind work that ultimately benefited Seth (and me).

In the early eighties, knowledge about risks and options was limited by a powerful orthodox medical culture and pharmaceutical industry that even today shields us from exposure to possibilities outside the conventional. There were many fewer options, and even fewer expectations. There was no Internet. We retrieved and compiled information differently than we do now.

In fact, there is a huge "alternative" world that includes mainstream medicine, like osteopathy, and unorthodox medicine—Ayurvedic for example—and the practice of various Eastern disciplines like massage, Yoga, acupuncture, and others.

The revolution in brain science legitimizes much that we once thought of as "alternative," and we see that the views of the experts are changing and expanding when it comes to some of these therapies.

Choose one issue in your life and examine how you think about it. Research alternative treatments and therapies and test your open mindedness.

We must be ready to take some risks to explore the efficacy of solutions. At the same time, we cannot jump at just anything in search of miracles. It's good to have an open mind but not so open our brain falls out.

I was no longer comfortable with the conventional approach to Seth's physical growth and I was no longer comfortable on my career path. *I began asking myself whether Seth's circumstance was a signal to me to reexamine the purpose of my life.* I pivoted, leaving behind my original aspirations to work in the theater and motion pictures.

I knew from the Feldenkrais workshops and my experience with Seth that I had a good touch. Many people suggested that I consider a career as a bodyworker or Feldenkrais practitioner, and there was a period of time before Haya was born when I seriously considered changing my career to bodywork. Weighing the pros and cons absorbed me whenever I had a break from the children and while I was studying all these new subjects.

The opportunity to write about my experience with Seth and the Feldenkrais method resulted in an article for *Family Circle* magazine. This event cemented the conviction that my mission was to bring a message to the world with words. Rejecting the idea of becoming a bodyworker, I began to devote myself to writing. This is when I wrote the first edition of *Uncommon Voyage*. I relinquished my hold on one career path and decided to venture down another. This is a story I have since heard repeated many times.

What opportunities or situations emerge when you are pursuing options for your child? How do they affect who you might become on this journey?

Try to remain open to embracing change. Our paths will rarely be etched in stone, and new opportunities might prove fulfilling. Research has proven that the children of mothers who tried harder to find meaning have better developmental outcomes.

I was studying subjects I never heard of never mind imagined exploring. People rolled their eyes and thought I was kooky. From personal experience and as a witness to what it meant for Seth as well as others, I felt compelled to share what I was learning. This is how I found out that not everyone wants to hear about what I learned and how I see things. I realize that "alternative" therapies or approaches are not for everyone and cannot remedy every condition; they do not mean the same thing to everyone.

The bottom line is to have an open mind; listen to information imparted by bona fide experts. Study is necessary. This helps us become more effective advocates for our child. When we become excited about the benefits and the positive outcomes and what we know to be true, we cannot help wanting to tell the world.

How do we share what we learn? What form does it take? Where and how do we tell others?

When we discover a solution that works for our child, we must not be surprised if we feel compelled to share it to benefit others. This urge may unfold as a new "calling."

I started out believing that the doctors—all those "acceptable" people—were my best chance at making things work—even when they were giving me conflicting opinions. Sometimes they were. What propelled me to explore outside the mainstream was drive and fortuitous events that put me in touch with unconventional options. I am not describing anything extreme. My personal challenges led me to find out more about "alternative" medicine including Feldenkrais and cranial osteopathy (not really "alternative") and Iyengar yoga.

Right after Seth's diagnosis I was way too scared to jump off into alternative waters. I knew nothing about alternative therapies and was hanging on to dear life to what was obviously accepted. Today there are more opportunities to explore options outside the mainstream.

The links between the body parts, the body and mind were real for me because I was immersed in work where their relationship was certain. If someone had just come and told me about all of this, I may have doubted them. What I was doing was lifting the limits off myself and off Seth. I was becoming a person who thought and wrote about subjects that were once outside my frame of reference; I did not even know they were there. It changed me.

It changed Seth. It changed our family. Without limits the future is wide open.

SUGGESTED READING:

Larry Dossey's book, *Space, Time, & Medicine*, altered my way of thinking about healing and medicine.

Thomas Hanna's *Somatics: Reawakening the Mind's Control of Movement, Flexibility, and Health* altered my thinking about what is "inevitable."

Chapter 9

ALL HANDS ON DECK

What you can do on your own right now.

"Faith sees the invisible, believes the incredible,
and receives the impossible."
—Corrie ten Boom

Touching my loved ones, my children and Jay, my close friends and family, frequently, casually, is natural to me. I held my babies close, carried them around until they were too heavy. A caress is usually my response to affectionate feelings. No one can touch—touch with all its meanings and in the greatest sense—like we as mothers can. Connecting to that capacity in ourselves connects us to those we love most and want to support.

My growing awareness from the Feldenkrais work was awakening me to the power of *my* touch—a mother's touch with healing intent for her son. The thoughtfulness I was learning in Carola's classes meant I put my hands on Seth with new attention. I was a serious student of Carola's "experiments" as she called them and the skills I was acquiring to stimulate my breathing translated into an awareness of Seth's breathing.

Touching acquired a new dimension after Anat quit New York and we knew she was not returning. I "took over the touching," which is how I literally put Seth into my hands. I took over. I used my ability from all I was learning to influence Seth's progress that summer. Every evening, when it was time for him to go to sleep, I took what Carola taught me and I sat on Seth's bed and quietly "worked" on his torso. I began at the base of his spine, on one side or the other, with what Carola called skinfold experiments.

Go through this chapter and pick two of Carola's breathing "experiments" one at a time. Try them for short periods on yourself and then with your child.

As your comfort level grows, expand the amount of time you perform one or another of the experiments. Introduce each experiment gently and for a brief time until you find how and what it elicits.

Skinfolding is one of the most impactful experiments I have ever known. It is an absolutely simple experiment and I recommend you begin here.

To experiment with skinfolding, gently gather your child's soft baby skin into your thumb and four fingers—do not pinch—lifting it ever so slightly away from its center. Hold it a moment until you see breath filling the space. Let the skin fall back toward your child's body. Rest. Repeat.

You can grasp the same skinfold several times. Or skip areas that are too tight to grasp easily and come back to them. If possible, work over one specific area for quite some time before starting on another fold.

When I rested my hand on the area where I had just taken a skinfold on Seth, I felt the softening reactions of his body underneath. I felt breath and blood come into that area. I worked over one specific area for a long time before going on to another.

I worked like this on Seth for at least half an hour every evening, always beginning where it was easiest, where there was the least tightness and the most suppleness. I tried to begin at the small of his back then work up from the rim of the pelvis to his shoulders.

Seth's responses were instant and dramatic. He wiggled and lengthened his trunk, yawning widely. Stretching out his entire body along the length of the bed, he inhaled hugely. He loved it. The skin is the largest organ of the body.

This was my nighttime experiment. At the end of half an hour his breathing was wide and steady. I could see the sides of his rib cage visibly expand, the breath filling out his entire torso.

On request I "worked on" Haya's friends, my nieces, and other family members. I never met anyone who does not enjoy this experiment. It feels unbelievably wonderful. "Cupping" is a method that the swimmer Michael Phelps uses and was much discussed during the 2016 Rio Olympics. Skinfold exercises are the layman's method of cupping. They both employ the same principle of separating the skin's prima fascia from the body and allowing the breath in—oxygenating the muscles and flesh.

In the daytime I incorporated many of Carola's other lessons into Seth's play. Tapping experiments were the easiest. Tapping influences the condition of the body immediately.

Gently tap your child's chest cage with your hand cupped slightly. Cover as much of his torso as possible, including back and breastbone.

You will feel your child's breath respond by deepening and widening.

When I tapped Seth, he had the same response I did when I tapped myself: he yawned and stretched and took deep breaths. I found this is the best way to wake a sleeping child. From that time forth, whenever I went to my children's rooms to get them ready for school or to wake them for any reason, I always tapped them lightly all over. They stretched and yawned, lengthened themselves, and arose with pleasure.

I did what Carola calls "pressure experiments" on myself and on Seth. I did this casually while playing with Seth and I made it a point not to make it "therapy."

Very lightly apply gentle fingertip pressure to the breastbone and the area between the ribs.

This is an experiment you can try on yourself; you may find yourself yawning and gulping breath quickly!

In Seth's case, the tightness around his rib cage and abdomen lessened, and an increased elasticity and softness enveloped him. I saw him sleep more calmly. I thought the clarity of his speech improved.

These subtle experiments had reverberations. There were no professionals, there was no formal therapy, yet these touches left him in a state of complete well-being. I felt empowered, knowing my actions were making a tangible difference in how Seth felt.

On rainy days we made cookie dough, and Seth helped me roll it out. Together we cut out the cookie shapes. These activities encouraged him to coordinate hand and eye movements. On the beach, while he was barefoot, I played with his toes and the soles of his feet. I rubbed his hands gently in the sand. If he was lying on his back, I played with him to mimic the movements I had explored in Anat's seminars. Whenever I could, I touched Seth around his diaphragm and rib cage as I learned to touch myself in Carola's lessons. I easily observed the changes in his respiration and the increased ease and softness that occurred in his body when I touched him like this.

When we were on the beach, I played imagination games with Seth: we lay on our backs and imagined that we were lying on a clear floor so we could see ourselves from below and above. Then we "painted" ourselves with black paint. We "painted" the length of our bodies, our legs, our arms—in our imaginations. Stimulating Seth's imagination was healing for him in his way and for me in my way. We were closely joined in these games and I could not help noticing how rolling and tapping and picturing affected me.

Seth loved these kinds of mind games, and we did many variations. During this kind of play I saw changes in his breathing—and mine! We played rolling games. Lying on our backs with our knees up, we rolled our knees from one side to the other. Sometimes we rolled all the way over, sometimes not. Or we counted.

I counted all the little knobs (vertebrae) on his back; he counted the knobs on mine. We rolled our eyes.

Choose a game that complements your child's abilities and impulses.

A very active child may seem best suited to an activity, like a rolling game and he also may appreciate an imagination game that calms his senses and allows his body to relax. Imagination games may be very freeing for an immobilized child.

Actual touching is involved in tapping and skinfold experiments. Other activities rely on imagination. These may be especially helpful for a child who is not as comfortable being touched.

Try these eye exercises that we did on the first days of the Feldenkrais training with Mia Segal:

Can you move your right eye to its corner? Back to center? Back and forth?

Can you keep your left eye still when you do this? Trace your eyebrows with your eyes. Slow and fast.

Make full circles with your eyes, slowly, now quickly.

Experiment. We each respond differently and with different abilities, but the actual experiments change us.

With all of these exercises and games, Seth had to be comfortable and find it fun, especially if it was coming from me. I wanted him to be at ease and feel what he might not have felt before.

Keep an eye on yourself and check any and all impulses to force or to become anxious about your effectiveness. These are games of discovery and must have no anxiety attached to them.

For you and your child to learn from these experiments, they must be comfortable. No forcing!

I was always talking to Seth, trying, playfully, to bring his consciousness to his body. I do not do this today, but there was a time that I always reminded him to soften his tongue, or to think about his big toe (read more about why these are important in the Appendix Tongues and Toes).

I was vigilant with Seth, encouraging many of the movements therapists taught me. I shaped play that invited him to develop more motor control. What I kept in mind at all times was the *fun* of it. From the Feldenkrais work and from Carola, I knew that being comfortable is the best state to be in for learning. Pain is a sense that something is wrong. I presented these exercises as games, as amusements. "Smile," I always told Seth. Be happy in the throat." These were things I learned in the Feldenkrais training. I continually repeated, "Smile."

Although we did not witness major steps when we first started these experiments—Seth was not suddenly standing up and walking around—we noted a significantly new freedom of movement and of naturalness.

More than anything, I felt connected to Seth. I was experiencing a new capacity in myself and loved my new relationship with my son. I was primed to expand my role in Seth's rehabilitation, to be more directly involved with his care and to be more in charge. Replacing a trained therapist over the long term was not my intention. I was simply reacting to my innate desire to bridge the space between therapists and the new sense of myself that was evoked in the meantime.

Science is absolutely corroborating the beliefs I held many years ago. In the November/December 2016 magazine, *WEBMD*, a study by the Cerebral Cortex journal cites evidence that shows how a mother's touch supports brain development. Researchers watched 5 year olds playing and recorded how many times their mothers touched them during playtime. Afterward, the children had a brain scan. Those whose mothers touched them most during the play session had stronger circuitry in regions of the brain related to socializing and mentalizing (the ability to understand your own and others' feelings, desires, beliefs and reasons for behaviors.)

Touching—taking in hand literally and figuratively—brought healing for Seth and for me because it was appropriate and perfect to the time, to his needs, and to mine.

SUGGESTED READING:

In my experience, Carola Speads is the master of this work. I was remarkably privileged to have been her student for those many years and recommend her book *Ways to Better Breathing* in particular.

The enduring concept of breath as healing continues to develop, and Belisa Vranich's new book—*Breathe: the Simple, Revolutionary 14-Day Program to Improve Your Mental and Physical Health*—holds much promise.

Chapter 10

SHIPMATES
Meeting the challenges for siblings
of special-needs children.

"All things change, nothing is extinguished."
—Ovid

As our lives and roles shifted when we became parents for the first time and shifted again with Seth's diagnosis, they changed when Haya was born. We were parents of two; Seth was a big brother. At the birth of Haya our mobile was reset to accommodate the needs of a newborn.

Seth's situation at any given time, however, was the mobile piece that determined much of Jay's, Haya's, and my experience. Each of us went through times when we felt left out or were overly concerned and there is still ongoing work to find balance as we age and change and find new ways to experience meaning in our lives.

Naturally, Haya's presence made a difference. We focused on our new baby and in the meantime there were no perceptible developmental gains for Seth. Everything was status quo, and I tended to let that be the fact until we could catch our breath.

When you think of your family as a mobile, what do you find are the particular triggers—positive or negative—that set you each in motion or knock you off balance? What specific actions help you achieve equilibrium?

If we identify and recognize how the rest of the family is affected by particular interactions, we prevent potential triggers from occurring and are better prepared if they do.

Haya seemed so grown up right from the day she was born. As she grew she spoke her mind at home and stood up for herself. She asserted her independence at a young age by tying her own shoes and dressing herself (things that were difficult for Seth to do for himself, although he eventually learned). In public she was quiet; shy outside of the house at least until she was more familiar with people and surroundings. Nothing felt out of proportion.

We assumed that Haya would simply accept what became our family's "normal." Then when Haya was four years old, I got a rude awakening. She started asking questions that stunned me. "Will Seth die from cerebral palsy?" "Is this going to happen to me? Why did it happen to Seth and not to me? "

I drew her close to me, held her, and answered as best I knew how—with the truth and with the information appropriate for her age. Haya acted reassured that I was responding to her, and was calmer. As she grew older, she asked different questions and so did her friends and other people.

In every instance I made sure to answer her truthfully. She

needed appropriate information. Andrew Solomon reports that "a diagnosis makes a huge difference to younger siblings who can use a simple explanation with friends; those with a sibling with no clear diagnosis struggle more."

What age-appropriate information do you provide the siblings of your special-needs child? When answering your child's questions, being truthful is of paramount importance.

As your child grows and realizes more, this is an ongoing conversation.

Considering Haya's place in the mobile helped me acknowledge and address Haya's special need: being the sister of someone with special needs. At the time there was little written about the effect on siblings who grew up in a family with a special-needs child. What I came to learn is that many children like Haya share similar characteristics, including compassion and patience. Children involved with a brother or sister with a disability often have better relationships with one another and other people. They must know that they have to be especially agreeable and pleasing. They also learn that difficulties can be surmounted.

Haya was quite reserved, which was a two-edged sword. It gave her more time to be observant and on the other hand, it betrayed a slight reticence, a hesitation. I worried that she hesitated out of fear of making a mistake—deep down I do not believe there are any. I believe—as does Jay—that knowing when to take risks and trust yourself is one of the more important lessons of life. We tried to strike a balance between encouraging her to take risks while maintaining the sensitivity she developed because she is Seth's sister.

Seth was used to being tested and rarely exhibited any anxiety about tests and, therefore, I didn't think twice when it was time for Haya to be tested for kindergarten. It turned out tests terrified Haya and she did not perform well on the standardized tests. Her scores implied she had below-average intelligence, which I could not believe and knew not to be true. The teachers and the head of school were as surprised as we were. (Literature about the siblings of special-needs children includes the possibility of this challenge of underperforming, but I did not know it at the time.)

We consulted the school psychologist, who observed that Haya often brought Seth into the conversation; she thought Haya compensated for him, worried about him. I had observed Haya's obsessive concern for Seth. The psychologist thought Haya's ability to take risks was being stifled because of her natural reticence. In addition, Haya was reacting with concern that she was outperforming her brother. In response, Jay and I began consciously to encourage Haya to risk more; encouraged her to express herself, and we did this by honestly expressing confidence in her. We also consciously praised and encouraged her to learn about herself— both her unique talents and the things that challenged her.

It seemed normal for Haya to have intense feelings about her brother's disability, as everyone else did—myself included. I had been concerned with Jay's feelings; my parents and my in-laws had gotten "special handling." I had to learn to do the same for Haya. We began consciously to encourage her to express her negative feelings (when she had them) so that they did not fester or build up inside of her.

What observations do you have about the behavior of family members—and others—when they are around your child with special needs? How do you spread your attention among your family?

When a family member suffers from a disability or from an illness, the entire family experiences it.

Whenever Haya concerned herself greatly with Seth's well-being, I thanked her and offered the reassurance that her father or I could be responsible for him. We did not want her to have any extra caregiving burden. Resentment and bad feelings toward a brother or sister with a disability are highest when a sibling has a lot of child-care responsibility. By involving Haya while easing her feelings of responsibility, we learned what studies confirm: *"a child with a disability has a positive influence on the lives of other children in the family"* (Lodewyks).

Sibling relationships make up one of a child's first social networks. Some of the potential negative effects siblings must deal with are embarrassment, resentment, and restrictions in social activity. Appearance and body image become increasingly important to teens. So is the appearance of family members. I saw the questions about Seth change as Haya and her friends grew older.

After school one day, Haya's friends were sitting around the kitchen table when Seth arrived home. As soon as Seth came in and began talking to me, the girls began to stare and get very quiet. Then they began to giggle and be silly. They started asking questions about why Seth talked a certain way and had trouble writing and doing fine motor tasks. Haya responded in a simple and straightforward way to their difficult questions. I steered the conversation to encourage a dialogue about valuing differences. Talking about it naturally set Seth, Haya, and the girls at ease while informing them.

What tools help you turn awkward social situations into opportunities for education, growth and understanding? How do you prepare for questions that require a truthful response?

Preparation is key. When we approach a charged situation with tools at our disposal, we direct its course while remaining calm, graceful, and more effective.

There existed an entirely other dynamic. Seth's mind was quick and agile and he was very skilled socially. Haya deferred to him in public spaces. If Haya expressed embarrassment or hesitation about performing tasks of her own, Seth's reaction often reassured her. In this way having a little sister gave Seth opportunities to care for someone else, when he had been cared for by others all his life.

Jay and I established family meetings when Haya entered elementary school. We realized the importance of having a safe place for each of us to express true feelings and an opportunity for the family to get together and agree—or disagree—on mutually important issues. Keep in mind the family meeting is not always holding hands and singing "Kumbaya." Each family has their own dynamic. It may involve raised voices, tears, and frustration. The important thing is the safe forum to express feelings about what is going on with each member as well as the family as a unit. The regularity of a family meeting provides structure and routine.

To prepare for the family meetings Jay and I took time for a few minutes of talking between ourselves and catching each other up on things the other might not be aware of.

Set up a regular family meeting and work with your partner beforehand to determine parameters—what will be addressed and the "rules of the road."

The more we as couples communicate at difficult times like these, the greater our collective strength, and the more ballast on a turbulent sea.

We are not always equipped on our own to organize and run a family meeting. Take advantage of resources. Don't feel you need to create this from scratch. There are low-cost (or no-cost) resources available for a structure that we along with our partner can use to put this useful experiment into action.

Haya was in kindergarten when she was left at home with Jay while Seth and I were busy with Dr. Frymann's treatments. We found that Haya reacted by arguing more with me and even Seth upon our return. We realized that she might resent Seth's having special time with me that she did not have. With that in mind I made it a point to dedicate time with her, one on one, just the two of us. We saw a change in her behavior immediately.

Carve out one-on-one time with your child who is not disabled—a time when she knows she is your main focus. This time can be brief but must be without interruptions.

Young children especially will react to our focused presence more so than to our words.

Like every other member of the family, each sibling swings back and forth between positive and negative emotions about her brother or sister. A child's piece in the mobile swings back and forth as its own entity—not just along for the ride—and our paying careful close attention to her needs is the best support we can provide. This attention helps a child reach her full potential in her own special circumstances, and brings equilibrium and balance to the family mobile, where each individual piece has a treasured place.

SUGGESTED READING:

Books about the experience of siblings of special-needs children were hard to find when I was raising Seth. Now there is a plethora, including treasures from Donald Meyer, such as *Views from Our Shoes: Growing up with a Brother or Sister with Special Needs* and *The Sibling Slam Book: What It's Really like to Have a Brother or Sister with Special Needs.*

I also love this book by Jeanne Safer, *The Normal One: Life with a Difficult or Damaged Sibling.*

Chapter 11

NAVAL ACADEMY

Accessing education and
appropriate services for your child.

"Arriving at one goal is the starting point of another."
—John Dewey

DISCLAIMER: *I am not an education expert; I am an expert on my child and our experience within the system. For this chapter, I called upon the expertise of Jean Mizutani[1] of* includeNYC. *I encourage you to read and consult experts to guide you. Work diligently, be involved; interview, make visits, observe, and take notes. Keep an eye on your child to see how he is reacting. Keep the faith that you **will** progress from fearful to hopeful in the quest to help your child fulfill his potential.*

School is not only about book learning. Early friendships are formed at school and children also learn to relate to adults outside

1. Jean Mizutani is currently the Senior Education Specialist at *includeNYC*, where she works with parents and professionals and conducts training on advocacy skills and special education. She is a key leader of *includeNYC's* Special Education Parent Center and participates in coalitions and advisory groups. Formerly a chef, she is the parent of a daughter with a disability. Jean first contacted *includeNYC* as a parent seeking help and volunteered for two years before joining the staff.

of their family at school. For a child with special needs, school is most often the place where he will receive services, including occupational, physical, and speech therapies.

School is also importantly a place of structure, and though schedules and philosophies may differ, each structure provides a framework vital for any child, especially those with special needs. Important choices dominate each stage on the education continuum, and when a child needs special education it is more complicated and even more important that we pay careful attention.

Many parents are in the midst of choosing a preschool or are in preschool when they first perceive differences in their child and decide to get a diagnosis. A child's nervous system is just forming in the beginning of life, and the developmental stages that coincide with two- to five-year-olds give parents and educators a chance to see—perhaps for the first time—the spectrum of a child's special needs. Preschool age often coincides with that particular developmental stage where delays and divergences become clear.

Early intervention is proven to be highly effective and most often high-quality services are best at early intervention and preschool points. These evaluations provide an objective description of our child, and are used to establish eligibility for services. Getting initial evaluations is critical even though they may make us nervous. They are also useful to measure progress once services begin.

Evaluations are needed to inform the meetings that will take place on a child's behalf (these IEP meetings are explained further below.) The evaluations must review each area of suspected disability or delay and may be from several different sources, both public and private. Parents who utilize the public evaluations can supplement them with private evaluations and information.

"What is the cost of the evaluation that is required?" "What does the education system pay for?" "What can you afford?" These are questions to ask for each evaluation. (In the *Storms at*

Sea chapter there is a discussion of some financial considerations.)

Most school districts will make available the tests needed to determine a child's aptitude and special needs. Depending on your financial situation, it is possible to enlist private psychological and educational experts to test and evaluate your child and make recommendations. When you use private testers, it is up to you if you want to share the results with the IEP team. It is a personal and strategic decision.

Find out everything you can to obtain the most accurate and holistic evaluation of your child. Determine what is covered financially by public resources and what you will need to budget for yourself.

Continue to use evaluations as a way of staying on top of how much your child is progressing and for getting what he needs at every stage. (Don't overdo it though!)

Use this chapter to become familiar with essential terms and acronyms that will help you. Get to know the "lingo" of special education. Learn the vocabulary and use the words. The glossary in the back of the book provides a good foundation, but it is important to go beyond by making connections and putting what you learn into practice.

Throughout this process, one of a parent's most important roles involves becoming an advocate for our child and paving the way for him to become an advocate for himself. Model this role for your child by taking it on whole*heartedly.*

Refer to what you learned about yourself in the *Home Port* chapter. Examine how it influences the way you guide yourself through the labyrinth of special education. Do you ask for referrals? Do you do personal research? Where and how do you keep the information? Do you keep track of appointments?

Develop attributes within yourself to call into service for you and your child in important situations like accessing services and other advocacy.

The Individuals with Disabilities Education Act (IDEA) says that "All qualified persons with disabilities within the jurisdiction of a school district are entitled to a free appropriate public education." (You will see this referred to as FAPE).

Your school or district (sometimes referred to as Local Education Agency, or LEA) will help you obtain initial evaluations. These evaluations are used to determine eligibility for special education services and to identify the services that are necessary to provide a student with FAPE. This step is part of the referral process for special education services, and parents are provided with information about their rights at the same time.

Parents should also ask for a copy of the "continuum of special education services" that lists all services and programs that are available. Although the LEA must be able to offer the full continuum, no one school is expected to have all programs and services. As a result, student placement is not necessarily limited to their local school.

Learn about the services that are offered in your local school district.

There will be a wide range of services around a wide range of disabilities.

The LEA is responsible for providing FAPE to all eligible students (although schools provide services, the LEA has ultimate responsibility). They have a commitment to help your child be a part of a school in your district (their first priority), or to authorize alternative specialized programing, either public or private. If a local education authority cannot provide a "free appropriate public education" through their continuum of contracted and approved services, there may be cases where parents can request funding for private school.

Identify the "players" or individuals who will be part of making decisions that affect your child.

Remember, you are one of the experts on your child. Keep this in mind during your search for other experts. Combine what they know with what you know.

Families with a child who has a disability need information about the disability itself, and also information about school services like therapy and other supports. Every state has at least one Parent Training and Information Center (PTIC) that provides this information. You will find the center for your state at the following link: http://www.parentcenterhub.org/find-your-center.

Ninety-eight percent of families depend on public education. Law dictates that a student is entitled to a Free Appropriate Public Education in the Least Restrictive Environment. Resources like includeNYC exist to help navigate the system; to help you be an effective advocate by providing resources for children, families and young adults with special needs including access and "love equity!"

As far as policy and the law: the starting point in your child's education is the assumption that your child—now the student—will go to the same school he would go to if he had no disability. This is only the starting point. It is necessary to weigh the pros and cons of a special ed school or specialized programs that may or may not be in your community or district. Rely on evaluations *and* your personal observations. Think it through. Take your time. Talk to other parents. Consult. Listen to others and listen to yourself.

At each step along our trajectory, Jay and I asked ourselves what was most important. We considered the school's philosophy, the class size, organization and location, space, groupings. No school meets every criteria so we picked what fulfilled most of them but also what "felt" right. We wanted Seth to get a great education with all the support and services we could muster while *keeping in mind that school and community go hand in hand.*

When researching programs for your child, seek a community that offers opportunities for him to meet people who he will like (and who will like him); somewhere safe yet stimulating and challenging.

Our comfort is very important at this phase; teachers and other families at school offer an important source of support and the opportunity for us to reciprocate support as well. We understandably want to be part of a community where we feel accepted.

A central component in the journey as a parent is how we convey information in our role as our child's advocate, and how and what we model for our child. (See the *Semaphore* chapter about messaging.)

Age-appropriate expectations are important. There are choices to make about school, about after school, about the relationship of special services to the school day: these are tough choices and they change. Stay involved and expect priorities and your child's needs to change.

Seek out parent groups within your school district or that hold regular meetings. In addition, look into the resources of online support groups and LISTSERVs that enable discussion. These groups may be hyper-local or specific in dealing with particular issues.

Connecting with other parents and knowing we are not alone goes a long way to buoy us.

When you begin meeting with key players like your IEP Team, there are some things to keep in mind so you will have as much of an impact as possible:

- Stick with the here and now. IEP meetings are generally once a year. Children receive academic assessments but are evaluated once every three years unless a request is made, in writing, sooner. In this way, plans can change as your child grows and develops and can address new challenges and recognize accomplishments.

- Know what you are asking for. For instance, are you requesting more occupational therapy (to hold a pen, use a fork and knife)? Or is an accommodation needed because you think your child needs more time in transitions or when taking tests?

- Be prepared. Rehearse. Work with family members or staff members at your parent information training center (PITC) and practice your role in the meeting. Imagine being one of the persons on the team and figure out how to be the best part of that team.

- Stay centered. Remind yourself what you are asking for so you stay focused and do not go off on tangents.

- Keep in mind that parents have recourse. There are always additional steps; nothing is out of the realm of possibility.

- Your child is a member of the team. If and when your child is able to communicate some of their own needs, you should expect and encourage him to attend the IEP meeting. At age 15, it is mandated that the student must receive an invitation to attend. Accept that invitation, even if your child can only attend for a few minutes at first, and gradually increase the time he participates. Your child's physical presence adds context and puts a face to paperwork and test results.

- Help your child advocate for himself. Your child's perceptions of his unique situation are crucial input for the child study team, and your role is to help them hear your child's voice as well as resources to help them represent themselves accurately and assertively. A good way to begin is by contacting and researching Kids As Self-Advocates (KASA). This national organization has many helpful links for both caregivers and children themselves, and can direct you to local resources.

One week after Seth started first grade, he stopped sleeping through the night. He got ornery at home and was always late in the morning. It took a while for us to tie the behavior to the situation at school.

When a child faces developmental challenges, look at factors that include what is going on at school, both academically and socially.

Discipline problems arise when a child is passed by in academics.

All along Seth's education continuum we made sure to get the necessary evaluations and to implement a variety of services. It is daunting, but know that you are not alone. Researching programs and learning to advocate for our child—and helping him become his own advocate—is hard work, it is true. However, the goal is to be surrounded by a community of teachers, families, and administrators where our child thrives and that means so do we.

SUGGESTED READING:

For the parents of preschoolers, I recommend you visit the Head Start website for a wide range of advice: https://eclkc.ohs.acf.hhs. gov/hslc/tta-system/teaching/Disabilities/families-too/Parenting/ disabl_fts_00044_081105.html

Because laws and resources differ from state to state, I encourage you to look online for the most current information. You will find many listed in the Resource Guide, and the following site is particularly pertinent.

"At a Glance: Free and Appropriate Public Education (FAPE)" at understood.org.

For the child moving into self-advocacy, KASA (Kids As Self Advocates) is an invaluable resource. Check out "Advocating for Yourself in Middle School and High School: How To Get What You Need" at fvkasa.org.

Dr. Brazelton's *Touchpoints* was my bible. For this reason I was aware when Seth was or was not meeting developmental milestones. In addition to his wonderful books, there are many resources at the following website: https://www.brazeltontouch-points.org/

Chapter 12

ANCHORS AND WINGS

Enlarging a child's world to encourage freedom and build self-esteem.

"A wise woman once said to me:
'There are only two lasting bequests
we can hope to give our children.
One of these is roots; the other, wings.'"
—Hodding Carter

There was more to Seth's life than therapy!

In his book *Helping Children Succeed: What Works and Why*, Paul Tough reports that the intervention that makes the most difference in children's lives is the encouragement of parents to play.

Tough found that children whose parents are counseled to play more with them did better throughout childhood on tests of IQ, aggressive behavior, and self-control. To improve children's opportunities for success, a powerful influence is the attitude and beliefs of the adults who surround them who play with them and let them play alone too.

Each child develops at his own rate, and as parents, we have our growth spurts and growing pains also. In our family we believed in hard work and we also considered play an important component of childhood—this period of exploration and innovation, learning and imagination. Whether a child is deaf, on the autism spectrum, or limited to a wheelchair, our responsibility is to create the circumstances that help him reach his optimal self. This includes time to imagine, to daydream, to wonder and to wander around in his mind.

When our child has the limitations of circumstance or accident that define "special needs," our role as parents is to seek the "work-arounds" that will help compensate for his challenges. A *work-around* enables a child with differences and special needs to accomplish a given task by innovating a solution. This is similar to the idea of an *accommodation* in special education—in some cases more time to accomplish the task, in others using additional tools to do so. Our work is to help our child figure out these work-arounds—a solution that is either such an accommodation or a situation where he will fit in. The focus should be on facing the challenge, not avoiding it.

As parents, it's good to use "aha" moments to improve and to learn. During one segment of the Feldenkrais Training I watched a videotape of Feldenkrais working and observed him bouncing children on his knee like they were riding horseback. This was one of my "aha" moments: the connection to horseback riding inspired me to explore opportunities for Seth to ride. I picked up on Feldenkrais' "message" about the efficacy of horseback riding.

What connections do you make to create opportunities for you and your child? Are you responsive to internal and external messages?

Be open minded: things we imagine are not available to us due to location or expense may be more accessible than we think. Keep at it.

When Seth was four, we worked out an arrangement for him to "ride" two or three times a week. Seth loved being on horseback. Immediately I recognized what Feldenkrais was demonstrating (and the powerful relationship between Yoga and riding). I understood why therapeutic riding has such a big presence in the world of special-needs children and adults.

Horses have been utilized as therapeutic aids since the time of the Greeks. The benefit of work with horses is not limited to those with physical limitations. Equine Assisted Therapy (EAT) encompasses a range of treatments that includes activities with horses and other equines to promote physical, occupational, and emotional growth in persons with all disabilities.

In riding (and yoga) the heels are rooted while the torso remains erect and at ease. The elbows are bent, while relaxed. The eyes are forward and concentrating. Pelvis, sacrum and head are in alignment. The interaction with the horse added to Seth's self-esteem. He learned to think of himself as tougher and stronger. Riding was good for him physically, mentally and psychologically.

Making the connection between the actions of Feldenkrais and something tangible I could get for my son reminded me how making connections opens doors.

During treatment sessions with Dr. Frymann, the only other person behind closed doors with Seth and the doctor was someone playing the piano. The doctor chose music sympathetic to her assessment of her little patient. As the sessions progressed, the music changed. Bach was always played at the close of a patient's sessions: "The perfect blend of science and art," the doctor said.

Dr. Frymann perceived the worth of music therapy more than seventy-five years ago and stated then that *music is primary for our well-being.* Today brain science proves music changes the mind. Over years the benefits of art and music therapy have acquired status among psychologists, therapists, doctors and teachers as activities that are healing and influential. The idea is to use creative activity as a vehicle for rehabilitation.

Music, dance, painting or potting—all are employed to soothe the mind. Today there are extensive resources, studies, and scholarly articles on the efficacy of creative arts therapy to treat and support developmental disabilities, depression, autism.

What activity does your child love to do that promotes his self-esteem and sense of independence?

Providing a protected space of safety and stability where a child flourishes encourages him to take risks and have adventures.

There are a great number of ways to help a child discover their interests. Teachers, doctors and therapists often have ideas. Or if we enjoy something (art, music, fishing) it is possible our child will find pleasure in it. This mutual pleasure holds the power to bring us closer to our child too. Remember, however, that eventually our child revises what knowledge we impart, challenging our wisdom and reshaping our values and we must learn to accept this.

Providing our child safe opportunities to take risks and explore is something we have to put front and center. Equally important, we are responsible for providing periods of silence to help him get to know himself and become familiar with his deepest feelings. This "active rest" does not mean leaving a child alone in his room for long periods of time that border on neglect. A child does not have to be busy all the time; he should certainly not be sitting in front of the tv or constantly playing with his phone. Letting a mind explore its inner world promotes knowledge and wisdom of self. It is about creative silence.

As grown-ups we must also model resiliency and demonstrate the ability to bounce back and to be resourceful. This encourages our children to be more creative by using what they have—or even what they don't have—to create solutions and make discoveries. Learning to navigate a disability early in life gives an advantage: disability is like any challenge or limitation: fundamentally human.

How can we use our limitations and teach our child to use his limitations as a path to self-discovery and exploration?

Limitations are a factor of life and must be used like we use gravity to walk on the earth. Without gravity we would all just float away.

To stay with the nautical concept, think of this: a vessel needs ballast to keep it centered and to keep it steady. A strong foundation in the family and a sense of self provides the weight needed for balance—balance meaning moving without falling over.

This stability implies equal or correct proportions. Proportional self-awareness and awareness of others is centering; it is ballast—a weight—that does not weigh us down.

Once we took a vacation that had no distractions (no television, no phone and we were living still in the age without internet so none of that!) We took walks, went swimming, played and sometimes talked, sometimes not. After a few days Seth began sharing some of his feelings of inadequacy with me; about being a "klutz." He described being slow and tired during the day and the details of his challenges in daily life at school.

By listening without judgement* I got important information from Seth, information that focused me on aspects of his life at home and in school and helped me make important decisions about his education and about rules at home. As Rumi says, "The quieter you become the more you are able to hear."

Practice active listening.[2*] Provide silences and learn how to work within these spaces to encourage your child to express himself.

Listening to what a child is saying rather than offering an opinion, advice, or an answer is our job as parents. Like observation, listening is a skill that needs to be developed and exercised.

Seth grew into his teens with a strong desire to see the world. As he grew more independent he took courses in the summer and

2* The US State Department offers the following guidelines for active listening: 1) seek to understand before you seek to be understood; 2) be non-judgmental; 3) give your undivided attention to the speaker; and 4) use silence effectively.

attended programs that supported his aspiration to prove himself. Some of these programs and activities required our diligent investigation to ensure Seth was safe while being challenged. As he grew older we advocated vigorously along with him to participate in challenging programs while focusing on the adaptations—workarounds—he needed for his circumstances.

Personnel in the various programs asked questions that sometimes felt tiresome and frustrating, but I would have been very suspicious had they not fully examined all the safety and health issues at stake.

It is crucial to make thorough investigations of programs. Write up or otherwise organize the questions requiring answers that pertain to your child's special circumstances. Make notes to review later.

Pay attention to how program personnel react to concerns. We must be secure that our child is safe and will thrive.

Seth's enthusiasm and determination prevail. He made it clear to the people he met then and the people he knows now how much he wants a particular program and how hard he will work to make it successful. This trait carried him through his education into his work life. He learned to be an advocate and to advocate for himself. Looking back, I give those programs credit for being open minded about Seth. It says a lot about an institution when they make accommodations and do so willingly. Of course, some institutions are organized and dedicated around activities for children with special needs. Seek them out.

Extracurricular activities helped mature Seth and give him confidence while becoming more realistic about his expectations for himself. That combination of confidence and awareness shaped him and us and helped us deal with the challenges that we confronted as each new school year unfolded and he moved further into the world as a young adult.

Keep in mind when our child takes risks—spreads his wings— we may feel as if we are left behind; we may not witness every growth spurt or great accomplishment. And it may not all unfold in a direct or a linear way either. The path is not a straight line, it is a spiral. Inherent in the spiral is elasticity and variability. Two steps forward, one step back. Progress is just that: a mixture. Putting on wings may mean shedding or losing something else. Try to relax. Use some of the techniques in the *Restoring* chapter to help you.

We give our child anchors so he is stable; we provide the foundation on which to take risks and explore. The anchor is the love of the family and a sense of security—a big enough sense of who he is (through silence and opportunities to express himself without being judged), to be confident and secure to spread his wings and soar.

SUGGESTED READING:

Founded in 1926, the National Association for the Education of Young Children (NAEYC) is a credible, wide ranging resource. On their site (naeyc.org) is research about the benefits of and links between play and learning.

For those readers interested in the benefits of riding, I put great stock in a book by Sally Swift, *Centered Riding*.

Chapter 13

STORMS AT SEA

Confronting universal challenges:financial
considerations, transitions of caregivers,
therapists, and doctors, and the place of faith.

*"To accept whatever comes, regardless of
the consequences, is to be unafraid. "*
—John Cage

Parents of a special-needs child have additional and different tests
than other parents. We must prepare and provision ourselves—
as much as it is possible—to weather the challenges. Universal
themes wind through the arc of our experience and they include
important issues like finances, transitions of those we depend
on—through death or otherwise—and the determination of the
place of faith in our lives. No doubt these issues impact the family
and each of us as individuals. If we acknowledge and address these
matters head on, we cope more effectively.

Financial woes are in direct proportion to the special need
of our child and the extent of our resources. However, rich or
poor the question remains the same: "How much does it cost?"
Whether it is long-term care or special schools and services or
transportation, money is an issue.

When Seth was first diagnosed, we started out with NDT-trained physical and occupational therapists, and after a sustained battle, our insurance paid a portion of the fees for these sessions. We jumped through hoops to get partial reimbursement for speech therapy and other medical needs. When we engaged Anat, no insurance company recognized the Feldenkrais treatments as eligible for reimbursement. (They couldn't even spell it!) To receive partial reimbursement for her sessions we saw a doctor willing to write a prescription for Anat's treatments at a small reduced cost to us. It was not easy but with Anat's help it got done. The question of a "pre-existing condition" was always an issue and we were constantly fighting with the insurance company. It was time consuming and did not always have positive outcomes. None of Seth's sessions with Charles or Carl Stough were reimbursed. We paid for these costs out of pocket.

There have been many changes in health care coverage and options since Seth was young; today insurance coverage varies based on company, policy, a child's condition, and the type of claim. Some will cover "alternative" or "integrated" therapies, and the Affordable Care Act may address pre-existing conditions and other circumstances to our benefit, but it will take some digging—diligence and digging.

Identify your entitlements from the insurance company, your locality, your State, and from the Federal government. Keep track of your questions and the answers. Maintain records of your expenses. Ask yourself if you need help with this. There are agencies and professionals available to guide you.

It is worth the time and effort to identify all available financial resources and professionals who can help us. We do not have to become experts if we can rely on a trusted advisor.

Scholarships are available for private schooling and there are some public funds available through the Carter reimbursement mechanism, a legal and financial process between families and their school districts. However, even if one qualifies, scholarships may not cover the full cost of tuition, and they may not be available to cover out-of-pocket charges for tutors and transportation. Tuition, tutors and transportation were our largest expenses during Seth's school years. Our "nest egg" became a fund we depleted to provide Seth with the education and the services that were best for him. It was worth it and we would do it again for sure.

Parents of special-needs children are faced with other financial considerations: the scope of a plan for our child's future. Our savings are not just set aside for our own retirement or a child's wedding; we are planning for another's lifetime.

As Elizabeth O'Brien wrote in the *The Wall Street Journal* in June 2016, "increasing lifespans make retirement planning more of a challenge for everyone—but especially for parents of disabled children." In her article she describes financial tools such as trusts and 529ABLE accounts and suggests the steps a parent can take while "planning for two lifetimes."

Family Voices is a comprehensive resource that "...aims to achieve family-centered care for all children and youth with special health care needs and/or disabilities." This organization provides a spectrum of information for families with special-needs children including issues related to finances and health care.

With the help of these resources, we take on the role of our child's advocate, possibly requesting needed services for a lower fee or asking for instruction for what we can do ourselves on behalf of our child until we can afford a particular therapy session, test, or treatment.

There is a reason I named this chapter "Storms at Sea." These issues are not easy. In most cases, our financial situation necessitates difficult decisions. With a finite resource, how to determine how and where to direct money on behalf of our child? The needs of each individual in the family have their own weight as well.

In developing a relationship with those providing care for your child, ask about payment options, including the ability to schedule sessions according to your ability to pay, bartering opportunities, and what you can safely and productively be doing with your child between sessions.

Discuss with your doctor or therapist select items from the Tongues and Toes chapter as well as the All Hands on Deck chapter. These no-cost interventions for our young child are possible solutions for dealing with lengthy times between visits.

For young people starting a family usually there is the expectation that our child will be able to surpass or at least attain our level of socio-cultural accomplishment. When a child has a special need it may mean finding social support from new or unexpected sources. "The birth of a healthy child usually expands a parents' social network; the birth of a child who is disabled often constricts that network" (Andrew Solomon quoting Alan Ross). We instantly belong to another community rather than the one we started in.

There is a sense of loss from our possible departure from previous social circles. It is helpful to get involved in groups that provide support and reach out to people in similar if not the same circumstances. Try to find another parent of a child with a disability. Some parents have chosen to be a parent helper. All over the world there are Parent to Parent Programs. The National Information Center for Children and Youth with Disabilities (NICHCY) has listings of parent groups. Get that information if you need it.

I resisted becoming a part of the "special needs" communities and fought hard to stay in the mainstream. At an appropriate time, I embraced an active leadership role in advocacy for children with special needs by getting involved with and eventually chairing the Board of Resources for Children with Special Needs, now includeNYC, which gave me a sense of acceptance and belonging in the special needs community. It is a fine balance and a matter of individual style, circumstance, and timing.

Many people who guided us through crucial early stages of Seth's development moved out of his life. There were transitions of individuals who Seth—and we—relied on for early intervention, for therapy, for the promise of a future of normalcy. Dr. Kessler relocated to the southwest within a year of our first consultation. Later Carl Stough, Dr. Breath, died. Dr. Frymann cut back her practice and we could no longer travel to see her. Most significantly, in Seth's childhood—on the cusp of his learning to walk—Anat left New York to practice out west. We reassured Seth that we could find someone else to help him. We girded him; we promoted in him belief in his potential. We remained calm in front of him. Behind the scenes I was up nights thinking and during the day I was on the phone networking. Seth trusted me and I was living up to his trust.

Transitions are a fact of life and a theme weaving throughout.

Our child with special needs requires special caregivers, and the community of people surrounding him is large. At the same time, people come and go. Therapists move away or stop practicing. Someone dies. Our child faces losses of those he has come to care for—presences in his life he relies on and is part of his routine. The transitions upset the structure of his daily life (and ours!).

A child grieves the loss of a significant presence in his life. As parents we grieve for our own loss *and* his loss. Adults usually have tools to explore feelings and weather the disturbances. It is up to us to use those tools on behalf of our child. We work through the loss to better reassure and guide him with his suffering. Being a part of his healing helps heal us. *All things are subject to change, and we change with them.*

The focus is on keeping an even keel—not rattled by these inevitable life changes. That depends on *modeling* resilience— pursuing the next iteration while being part of creating it.

Examine how you handle transitions for yourself. What example do you set for your child when a therapist moves away or in the face of other transitions that are inevitable?

Send the message that you trust yourself to get what is needed. Send that message to your child and to yourself! What our children see reflected in us sends the most important message to them.

Seth understood that Anat and others were gone but that *I remained.* I was the rudder, the constant; I had been all along and

I would continue to be. I was always there: interviewing, coordinating, distilling, and overseeing.

There is always the possibility of loss. One way to facilitate transition is to expand the relationship between the therapist, teacher, tutor, doctor beyond the room and beyond the moment: incorporate into our life the important messages and lessons our doctor or therapist is conveying. We have to accept the responsibility of being taught. Becoming good students is ultimately up to each of us.

What motivates a child to be a good patient or learner? What drives him? Curiosity, our own respect for learning—each of these contributes to how a child becomes a good student. The lesson is learning how to take what is taught beyond the treatment room or the treatment table and into the world. This is how we learn what learning means. If we take the lessons of our teachers and incorporate them into our life, our teacher never truly leaves us.

The transition *into* a relationship presents challenges as well. For instance, Seth put up resistance with Anat (and later Frymann) in the very beginning and, yet, when he "caught on" to the meaning of what was happening for him, and after he had tested and explored, he organized himself for his sessions and in fact, never complained about going. Later this was true about Dr. Stough who he went to see regularly without complaint and eventually on his own as he grew older.

On the other hand, from the time he was sixteen months old and throughout the two years of treatments by the speech therapist, Seth was never compliant. He voiced discontent and refused to practice anything she taught him. At the time I wasn't listening to these messages from Seth. I was desperate to "fix" everything I could.

Observe over time your child's responses to therapists, to therapy, to doctors and teachers. Learn when and how to motivate your child to be persistent; learn when to cue him and when to take his cue!

It is a fine line between obstinacy and real discomfort and it is important to decipher the discrepancies; what might just be a "bad day." Know your child.

Enduringly is the subject of our grief. In all our stories as parents there is rejoicing and there are elements of grief and loss. It is a different kind of grief being the parent of a child with special needs from the grief brought on by the death of a child or loved one. Our child is not gone. He is right there demanding a lot of care and attention. Our feelings are complex and ambiguous when we mourn the loss of what our child might have been—or our life might have been—while at the same time struggling to care for the child who is in the life we have. Our grief may show itself in feelings of despair, anger, and possibly bitterness. We cannot be afraid to show emotion; we work to maintain a positive outlook as we stay in touch with reality. Success has to do with our coping skills. Taking care of ourselves and keeping daily routines as normal as possible reinforces those skills.

We can begin by learning to cope with the dissonance between the image we had of our child and the reality of our child. We say that our struggles ennoble us, but we do not know who we would have been without them. We might have been equally wonderful. By finding a place to tell our story, we can take ownership of our narratives including our individual challenges and accomplishments.

Make a timeline of life. Retell—to a trusted friend or in writing—the birth story of your child and the major milestones you faced and worry about facing.

There is a lot of grief in living out the logistics of our lives; we need time to feel and make room for mourning. The Restoring chapter provides some tools for replenishment.

When faced with the needs of our child, some of us find our faith shaken; others find it a source of strength. Either path is healthy as long as we allow ourselves to ask difficult questions, brave challenging solutions, and embrace the change before us. How can we connect with the strength inside ourselves? There are a few possible tacks to take. One positive source of strength and wisdom is a minister, priest or rabbi; a good friend of a counselor. Seek those who have shown strength for you before in your life. Find new sources if needed.

Throughout my experience of Seth's childhood there were instances that tested me. I found myself presented with a choice, and choosing faith provided me with a strength to go forward. For example, once Seth had an accident on a holy day in the Jewish calendar and that coincidence forced me to think about my emotional life, the life I experienced as a wife, a mother, a parent of a special-needs child through the lens of that particular holiday—a holiday that emphasized atonement, forgiveness, and renewal.

That night in my personal journal I wrote that when Seth was born, I had no idea that being his mother would take me on this journey. Of course we never know where life will lead us. What I recognized was that the spiritual phase of my passage had taken hold. I seized the opportunity and rededicated myself to remaining attentive to life's lessons and turn them into opportunities for learning and growth. I committed myself to trust in the power of daily practice even when I might not always understand it, feel like it, or even wonder why I am doing it. This remains an enormous source of strength for me.

One place where we felt accepted as a family and Seth was accepted for himself was our house of worship. For that matter we got more and more involved, eventually becoming an integral part of the community. The children made friends there. We made friends there but, mostly, it was about carving out regular, weekly, consistent time that was about us as a family. The regularity of it was dependable. It expanded our sense of time. We obeyed the commandment, "Remember the Sabbath and keep it holy," which was a way we learned to consecrate time; to recognize how sacred it is.

Consider the role of a community of belief—whether it is religious or secular—where you celebrate life's joys, receive support in crisis, and come together with your child and family.

Sometimes the faith of our childhood provides a source of strength for us as adults. Sometimes the discovery of an ancient practice or learning meditation is a path to peace.

Although our children grew up in a big city with all the "noise" of urban life, each of them found their individual voice.

We learned to make the quiet spaces, intimate time to hear that voice. And for all of us to hear each other.

What "Sabbath" do you have in your week? Find or create a regular time for ritual and rest that you celebrate as a family.

Sabbath can be Friday night, a Sunday or Wednesday morning. It is about creating space for the consecration of time—a space where what happens is unpredictable yet healing.

In such spaces everything and anything can happen; can be remembered; can be felt. It is not always so easy. In the quiet sometimes I fall into blaming myself for not being more, knowing more, especially at the beginning. For instance, by then I had recognized the importance and value of early intervention and faulted myself for not getting help for Seth sooner. Early intervention is key—pivotal—to making big differences. I did the best I could, learning as fast as I could. I wish I found Dr. Frymann in the first months, day or hour, but we do what we can with what we have at the time.

Focus on finding peace. Find a space for thankfulness in the present moment. Accept all the feelings, the good with the bad. How are you containing—embracing together—"mixed emotions?"

Let go of regret. The only thing you get when you look back is a stiff neck.

Parents often need help adapting. According to Alan O. Ross in *The Exceptional Child in the Family,* "...they often need help in adapting their behavior to the reality—they must learn to cope with the dissonance between their image of 'a child' and the reality of 'their child.'" It has to do with parents' coping skills, dynamics among healthy members of the family, and the importance parents place on how people outside the family perceive them. Ross wrote that children of mothers who try harder to find meaning have a better developmental outcome. When we are searching for meaning for ourselves it doubles in importance because *it is helping our child.*

SUGGESTED READING:

Both of the following books are highly recommended by a variety of websites and were referenced by the "Wall Street Journal" in July 2016:

Hal Wright's *The Complete Guide to Creating a Special Needs Life Plan: a Comprehensive Approach Integrating Life, Resource, Financial, and Legal Planning to Ensure a Brighter Future for a Person with a Disability.*

Peggy Lou Morgan's *Parenting an Adult With Disabilities or Special Needs: Everything You Need to Know to Plan for and Protect Your Child's Future.*

Chapter 14

RESTORING

Drawing on life experiences for the tools to restore yourself.

"The wise don't expect to find life worth living; they make it that way."
—Anonymous

Like the chapter All Hands on Deck, this chapter offers concrete suggestions to help deal with what life is throwing at you. I encourage you to read and consult certified practitioners to guide and support you. For this chapter, I called upon the expertise of Vince Corso[3] of* Compassion Identity *to provide exercises and insight.*

In addition to specific medications and therapies to "treat" a person, life experiences and situations hold the potential to provide healing. For me, Haya's birth and the fact of being Seth's mother—though each presented challenges—were healing

---

[3*] *Vincent M. Corso, M.Div., LCSW-R, is a licensed clinical social worker who worked for Visiting Nurse Service of New York Hospice Care for almost twenty years developing their landmark Bereavement Program. Currently Vince is developing* Compassion Identity *to promote the concept that self-awareness is vital in order for a person to better serve and work with others.*

forces and helped me grow into and accept the person I am.

For every parent, each new situation and new doctor/therapist appointment usually means recounting a child's birth story, a description of the diagnosis (or hearing it cruelly repeated) and the child's symptoms. In the beginning it was hard for me to face the facts of my birth experience—Seth's birth experience—to acknowledge the factors that contributed to Seth's cerebral palsy because of my agony about that night of labor.

Coming to terms with my experience of Seth's birth and recognizing and accepting the consequences for Seth—to the extent that we could know what the consequences were going to be—was a gradual process and is ongoing.

Our role as a parent means we are a witness and storyteller while also a character in the story. At many junctures we have feelings about our child's circumstances and the role we play— positive and negative. Examining and exploring our feelings helps *us* separate how we feel about our child from how we feel about his diagnosis or situation. This is important when answering questions and filling out forms. Remember that a clear and dispassionate description of facts allows a doctor or therapist to do their best for our child.

I was calm while I was pregnant with Haya, knowing Seth's circumstances were not a result of a preexisting condition or a problem with my pregnancy. After Haya was born, however, I was unprepared for the contrast between my two children and how it made me feel.

Haya's body *felt* different than Seth's. Hers was pliable and soft where his had been—and still was—stiff and brittle. Because of this I was split between joy and grief during Haya's milestones. Had she been my first born and had I touched her before Seth was born, I would instantly have known that something was wrong with Seth. I remembered how the massage therapist who handled

Seth as an infant tried to alert me to the stiffness in his body. Eventually experience revealed that an osteopath would definitely have also known there was something wrong.

The comparison between Seth's development—or lack thereof—and Haya's "normal" development was extreme, and it was in front of me every day. It was difficult. Over the course of that first year I had to touch the sorrow I had never given into after Seth's diagnosis. Mixed into the joy and ecstasy of Haya's birth and the expansion of our family was a touch of grief, fear, and self-doubt.

I had to forgive myself for not knowing more and doing more in the last months of my pregnancy with Seth or on the night of the birth or for being ignorant in the first ten months of Seth's life about what was happening. I had to forgive myself for not heeding the words of those like the massage therapist, for not introducing cranial osteopathy earlier. Absolving myself allowed me to weave purpose from those occurrences and learn that thoughts of regret served no useful purpose. As Admiral David Jeffries stated, paraphrasing Pat Schroeder, "You can't roll up your sleeves if you're wringing your hands."

Mourn. Ask yourself, "What did I hope for?" Express and describe, preferably in writing, what you may have _imagined_. Write about the shape of the hopes and expectations you had as you prepared for your child.

This is a very unique, personal, and individual journey. Approach it a little at a time and give yourself permission to go slow.

Comparisons between what we expected and our current reality—or between our special-needs child and their sibling or other children—may bring feelings of sadness and frustration. Practice letting go of what you cannot change and focus on each child individually while celebrating being a family. Know it is natural to have feelings about the health/development of other children including their siblings as compared to our child with special needs.

Create a ritual for ridding yourself of what you cannot change and bringing to light what there is to celebrate.

Consider deleting what you wrote about your unfulfilled hopes by tearing it up, burning it, or otherwise erasing it.

Once we have allowed ourselves to release the past, release regret, our arms are open to embrace the present and *be* present to our reality.

Celebrate "What do I have?" Detail the unique joys and gifts that your child represents and possesses. Plan a commemoration to appreciate your child.

This celebration can be part of a child's birthday or a holiday celebrated each year. Display in your home a special image or symbol that represents the gift your child is to your family. It is healing.

The process of caring for oneself is experienced differently by each of us, as is the need to do so. Some of us feel a physical ache or longing. Others of us feel uncharacteristically distracted, unable to concentrate at work, home or school. Still others question the purpose of life itself, and enter a time of spiritual darkness. Most of us feel as if we are on a wild roller coaster ride, one minute feeling calm, the next feeling upside down.

When we give ourselves permission to feel and we pay attention, we become *self-care seekers*. We allow ourselves to *re*create or *re*generate our current circumstances or perhaps even discover a new one. When we imagine a reconstructed view of the future, we more easily embrace new opportunities for growth and relationship. Many of us accomplish this work quite well.

Self-care seekers have the necessary tools within or around themselves (family, friends, time, a spiritual life or personal philosophy) to accomplish the work of self-care. Acknowledge that this is indeed work and requires regular practice. Trust in the power of daily practice even if you might not always understand it, feel like it, or even wonder why you are doing it.

Though self-care is challenging work, we accomplish it by accessing our personal inner resources. If the task becomes too heavy to handle alone, we can seek out others who are able to assist us and walk with us on our journey to wholeness.

- **Recognize the loss:** Knowing means feeling and holding the pain.

- **React:** Experience the emotions that are yours.

- **Recollect:** Reflect on what was and on what could have been.

- **Relinquish:** Once the foot touches the path, the journey moves forward.

- **Readjust:** The picture of "what is" takes on greater clarity and purpose.

- **Reinvest:** Self-awareness opens new vistas allowing us to love in new ways.

Here are some signs to help us know when to seek out additional support:

- Are we experiencing an ongoing sense of numbness or isolation within ourself or from others?

- Are we highly anxious most of the time? Is our anxiety beginning to interfere with our relationships, our ability to concentrate or our day-to-day functioning?

- Do we feel that we are continually preoccupied with the root cause of our anxiety?

- Are we afraid of becoming close to new people for fear of experiencing rejection or misunderstanding?

- Are we taking on too much responsibility for needy family members or friends? (What constitutes "too much responsibility" may vary greatly and depend on the situation, but if we are feeling heavily burdened, angry or feeling "suffocated," it might be time to speak with someone.)

"Finding our way through grief is a lot like making a tapestry. As we grieve, memories of the past—of our losses—are gradually being gathered up, reclaimed and woven into the present. Eventually a pattern emerges: a picture that shows the past and present have been rewoven.

To appreciate the art of tapestry is to look at it from both sides. The back of the tapestry can tell us about brokenness. There we can see where all kinds of broken threads were left dangling and where they were securely tied together again.

When we study the front of our tapestry, we see something quite different. We see the bigger picture. We see the connections. We see the unique patterns and shapes of our life has created. We might see a wholeness—that there is beauty. That in grieving our losses we have become artists of life."

—Donna O'Toole

Practice   Silence
Rest   Listen
Reflect   Respond
Resolve

SUGGESTED READING:

During difficult passages I often return to Pema Chodron's books, especially *When Things Fall Apart: Heart Advice for Difficult Times.*

Meditation is a safe and simple way to balance personal, physical, emotional, and mental states. It is easily learned and is a proven aid to dealing with stress. Sharon Salzberg explores this in her book *Real Happiness: the Power of Meditation: a 28-Day Program.*

LIFESAVERS
Ten tried and true moorings to latch on to.

Simple measures can be profoundly effective.

TOUCH YOUR CHILDREN
Touch is the great sense.
It is touching; it touched me;
I touch the stars when I am with you.
It is important to know *how* to touch and
to know how much we communicate with touch.

MAKE EYE CONTACT
Look into your child's eyes.
Look often.
The eyes are our active seekers
of the essence of life.

ENCOURAGE MOVEMENT
Movement is learning.
Run, swim, play, roll—it moves me, we moved,
they were moved.
Moving lets the brain know where the body is
in relation to the world.
Motion is the number one function of structure
and it is the root of psychological functioning.

OBSERVE WELL
Trust what you see: it is the truth.
Use your eyes and ears and trust your heart.
Sucking, crying, laughing, sleeping, eating—
how does your baby/child seem to you?
Develop your powers of listening and seeing.

"TALK" WITH YOUR CHILDREN
Talking with a child helps him explore his feelings and
express himself. Talking means dialogue—
asking questions that cannot be answered
with a simple yes or no.
Be sure you are listening and are open to your child's
verbal and nonverbal responses.

FEED YOUR CHILDREN WELL!
(while sitting and eating with them)
Good nutrition is the best prevention against ill health,
and equally important to what you eat
is when and how you eat.
Mealtime is a social time, a time of conversation, interaction, and a chance to listen and observe.
Involve your child in preparation.

LEARN TO PRACTICE
AND TEACH YOUR CHILD TO PRACTICE
Practice anything:
piano, swimming, drawing, meditation, chess,
 a language, cooking
and then try to do it every day.
The habit of practice is nourishing—
practice breeds strength and discipline, perseverance, and
the ability to be free of old patterns and silly mistakes.
It gives feedback—
a deeply satisfying sense of yourself.

KEEP GOOD RECORDS
Record-keeping is like marking a trail;
it safeguards memory.
Write it down, save it, and make files that are well labeled
and organized.

GET EDUCATED

Do not hesitate to ask every question
for which you need an answer.
Ask your doctors whatever you want to know—
do not hold back.
Information is not always outside of yourself.
Combine what you know inside
with the information you acquire outside.

TRUST YOUR INSTINCTS

You know more than you think.
That old adage, mother knows best, is true.
We have to believe that what we know counts.
Those wise voices inside of us
are our most important guides.
Do not expect miracles
 but remind yourself that miracles happen.

SUGGESTED READING:

Adele Faber & Elaine Mazlish have written a series of books since coming out with the original *How to Talk so Kids Will Listen & Listen so Kids Will Talk*. Choose one depending on your child's age or level of development.

Some consider "discipline" a bad word, but in the context of this book it is about providing structure for our children. *Discipline the Brazelton Way* by T. Berry Brazelton and Joshua D. Sparrow.

AFTERWORD

Within the commonality we share as parents of a special-needs child, we each have singular stories to tell. In *Uncommon Voyage* I told my story and I presented tools for you to find your voice and tell yours.

It's good to forgive ourselves our mistakes and our shortcomings and go forward one step at a time like the way Seth learned to walk: one step at a time. One step at a time is the means to solve problems. As much as possible we use what comes into our life taking one experience into the other, learning how to throw our emotional arms around whatever happens.

In the *The World According to Mister Rogers*, Fred Rogers says,

Part of the problem with the word "disabilities" is that it immediately suggests an inability to see or hear or walk or do other things that many of us take for granted. But what of people who can't feel? Or talk about their feelings? Or manage their feelings in constructive ways? What of people who aren't able to form close and strong relationships? And people who cannot find fulfillment in their lives, or those who have lost hope, who live in disappointment and bitterness and find in life no joy, no love? These, it seems to me, are the real disabilities.

Someone smarter than I am once said the reason Seth is among the chosen is that he came into the world knowing what he "owes," and the rest of us have to wait to find out. We are all temporarily abled or temporarily able bodied; we all impact the mobile that shifts in our direction at times. In the family a special-needs child is the mobile piece that makes the most demand on the mobile's fulcrum, and the other pieces take shape and position in response.

My marriage to Jay has had ups and downs like any long-term relationship—it's a marathon. We help each other by balancing responsibilities, by trying to respond to each other with thoughtfulness, awareness, caring. We had our moments; about Seth and Haya we worked hard at being in sync (this remains a work in progress).

Seth and Haya's relationship is also very complex and possesses a dimension that I do not observe in other siblings. To me, this dimension contributes more than any other fact to their lives, to the people they are, and to the people they are becoming. Their relationship with one another defines each of them and how they interact with others and with the world.

I changed when our son came along. I am not who I used to be. I am rarely angry that Seth's life has the challenges it does. When I grieve, I am also grateful—grateful that he is different because we see life through different eyes because of him. I am more because of Seth. I am more than I ever knew I could be. I am thankful we do not take small moments for granted. I am grateful that every triumph is just that—a victory. I am going to look back on my life and know I drank in every moment and soaked up our life, the good and the bad.

Jay and I each had plans when we prepared for the birth of our baby boy so many years ago. In his mind, Jay was tossing balls to Seth. I had not imagined carrying my son around until I couldn't anymore. We created new dreams and new hopes based on our new reality. Seth became who he is today because of his limitations—true for all of us. Limitations are our gravity.

Seth had the dream to ride a bike and he tried really hard to learn. It didn't happen. Since he couldn't ride alone, we learned to ride tandem. We found a way to make it work and we did so together. We morphed. Now that Seth is an adult, the same is true in the parts of his life that have nothing to do with me: he finds a way and he maps his own course.

The decisions we made in Seth's early life—especially when we were in control—set a course for his voyage to adulthood. Some of the concerns we had then are nearly obsolete now. We wondered if Seth would drive a car. He does with some limitations, but it is no longer an issue in the sharing economy and with the advent of self-driving cars. It goes back to the word *handicapped*. This word is best reserved to describe a disabled person who is "unable to function" owing to some property of the environment. Thus people requiring a wheelchair may or may not be handicapped depending on whether wheelchair ramps are available to them. Today and into the future innovation and technology are making a big difference to people with "handicaps!"

At the heart of things we must not look for quick fixes. We cannot make gods out of humans. We cannot look only outside of ourselves for answers: the search is an ongoing process inside of ourselves *and* outside of ourselves.

Wellness encompasses everything: our habits, our thinking, our attitude and our commitment. *Holistic* can be assigned to all functions of parents, doctors, teachers, coaches—are we using a "wholeness" model? Does this model encompass wholeness in the most profound sense, with nothing left out? Essentially, do our actions enable us—enable this child—to function optimally, whatever that is? And is it enabling me, us, the family to function at our greatest potential?

The more we push ourselves outside our comfort zones, the bigger our comfort zones become. When those zones are bigger, our emotional self is larger, our intellectual capacity is stretched, and we are more able to live in this world without fear and with courage. Risk is built into life. A life ruled by fear is not living. The only failure is not trying.

Raise your sails.

APPENDIX:
TONGUES AND TOES

This Appendix explores what I learned off the main course. Open your mind. Explore. Take a few risks.

*"The natural force within each one
of us is the greatest healer of disease."*
—Hippocrates

*"Why not go out on a limb?
Isn't that where the fruit is?"*
—Laura Shapiro Kramer

The structure of the body is intimately related to the way it functions. The trauma of being born is the most common cause of structural problems in babies and Seth's birth was certainly a trauma.

Dr. Frymann taught that how a baby sucks and swallows indicates how the area at the back of the head—the occipital artery—is affected by the stress or the degree of compression that is sustained as the infant is pushed through the birth canal. Vomiting—spitting up—and sleeping are other accessible factors to examine for structural clues.

The principle is always the same: the body functions as a whole, not a series of isolated, independent parts. The signs are easiest to read in the newborn because a baby's nervous system is basic. We just have to trust what we "see."

The movements involved in our actions affect every other aspect of our organism. There are consequences to *everything*. Everything matters.

Expand your vocabulary. As we parent it is important to learn all the words! In the case of special needs, there are many more words we need to know. Our parenting experience is like going to a foreign country. We have to learn another language. We must be open to the "culture" and learn the ways and means.

Seth's sensory experience—as is the case with many individuals with cerebral palsy or other special needs—is vastly different from our own but we certainly learn as much from him as he benefits from what others know. Be open minded—but not so open minded that your brain falls out!

THE BIG TOE

During one segment of my Feldenkrais Training we were focused on our feet. Of course during the training we were always barefoot; like Anat and like Iyengar, being barefoot is the conduit to sensory growth and information.

In class we were exploring the stages of human development and we discovered sitting up is integral to the action of the feet! We played with using the big toe to paw the ground, rubbing it along the floor where we worked. We realized we could not roll ourselves over from our backs and propel ourselves up to sitting without an action of the big toe!

One rainy weekend afternoon I was at home lying on our bed with Haya when she began stroking her big toe over and over again along the bedcover. The repetition was unceasing. All of a sudden Haya sat up. It was exciting. I was witnessing the normal developmental process.

Seth never sat up like this and Haya's development telescoped Seth's limitations. (The work in the Training underscored the resounding subtleties of differences between my two children.) Seth never used his big toe to progress along the normal path of development. He never sat without assistance; he needed to be set into position or be propped up. To this day it remains very difficult for him to get up from the ground. For eighteen months after the diagnosis he never even felt his big toes on the ground because he was wearing the *inhibitory* casts. Thankfully, Anat insisted we remove the casts and she and other professionals used his big toe to stimulate him.

When he was young and I went to the dentist with Seth I helped him relax through his big toe! If he was tense or 'spastic' and had to hold his mouth open, it instantly produced a gagging reaction in him. I sat nearby and said, "Relax the big toe, Seth. Just keep your toes soft." It worked! We had to keep at it, reminding him, focusing him and helping him recapture the feeling but the effect was dramatic. (Mind over matter!)

In Iyengar yoga, "join the big toes" is the first direction at the beginning of every standing class. Senior yoga teachers have told me the big toe is the conduit to the inner groin, and, therefore, the entire basis of the action of the spine.

THE TONGUE

Like the tongue, the big toe is significant. As Anat emphasized thirty years ago: bare feet and a limber tongue! The tongue has genuine power and influence. This is a fact that is only partially recognized and rarely discussed. It is a fleshy, movable, muscular organ. It is often at the center of function, especially movement. It attaches to the floor of the mouth and is the principal organ of taste, an aid in chewing and swallowing, and our primary organ of speech. Dr. Frymann told her students that the first thing she asks parents is, "How did the baby suck?"

In Chinese medicine when you go to see the doctor the first

thing he asks you to do is to stick out your tongue so he can look at it because the tongue reveals what is going on *inside* the body.

Our sympathetic nervous system consists of two large nerves on either side of the vertebral column. All these nerves have their roots coming out of the thoracic and lumbar regions of the spinal cord. She taught that it is important to know that the hypoglossal nerve that innervates the tongue, passes between the basilar and the condylar parts of the vertebrae.

As Thomas Hanna writes in one of his numerous and lucid essays, "We must think of ourselves as being controlled not from without but from within." What is more within than the tongue? In Mr. Hanna's view we have from birth until death a loop of four elements: skeleton, muscles, nervous system, and environment. I believe the tongue links all of these elements.

Anat put a lot of emphasis on Seth's tongue. She wanted him to practice putting the tip of his tongue into both corners of his mouth where she dabbed applesauce, something he loved passionately. If he failed to cooperate, applesauce was prohibited at home.

CRAWLING AND CROSS PATTERNS

In a lecture Dr. Frymann and Dr. Springall presented—The Developmental Process of Children with Special Needs—the doctors pointed out the strong correlation between how much a child progresses in individual stages and a child's long term intellectual development.

They emphasized that children who miss normal developmental processes do not function as well as the children who do pass through normal stages of development. Frymann taught that the brain is a complex computer that is not programmed at birth. The organization of the central nervous system does not happen automatically. Plus there is a direct correlation with development and a longer process of trial and error.

Sensation and motor ability are vital to the programming of function. Each stage in a child's development is essential to the development of the next stage. Each stage in the human individual, even on the cellular level, recapitulates the prior stage. Development can be viewed as an ever-expanding spiral (and this is true in every realm: spiritual, emotional and physiological). Random floor movements and then crawling on his/her stomach and finally cross-lateral crawl—all this brings physiological changes to the brain.

As a child moves along the widening turns of the spiral, there occurs a return to various developmental themes, but each time these are experienced, it is with a broader perspective, with new knowledge, new skills, and greater independence.

Seth returned to Dr. Springall for reevaluations. The doctor was pleased with Seth's progress and modified Seth's exercise programs so that Seth would be simulating cross patterns and "digging in more with the big toe." (I laughed to myself.)

By engaging in a program of exercises designed especially for him, Seth was stimulating and reorganizing his central nervous system along the normal developmental spiral and he achieved more control over himself. He practiced on his own at home twice a day.

The exercises simulated crawling and cross patterns of creeping. Dr. Springall believed that Seth's reading would develop more quickly once he began doing these exercises. He turned out to be right.

Most of the objectives in the exercises involved the big toe and cross patterns! The doctor wanted Seth's big toes to drag on the floor during one part of the simulated crawling exercise.

Doctor Springall suggested we get a special keyboard for Seth's computer, a device that he thought would help to further enhance the cooperation between the two hemispheres of Seth's brain. He also encouraged us to emphasize skills that did not rely totally on the visual process.

DAILY LIVING

During his teens Seth asked for a way to learn how to do some of the daily tasks that we take for granted but challenged him enormously, such as tying his shoes, buttoning his buttons, cutting up his meat, pouring from a pitcher.

We found an occupational therapist, who took Seth on as a student for a limited number of sessions. Seth learned to tie his own shoes, cut his food with a knife alone, not easily, but successfully, and he acquired a small tool to help him with buttons.

THE EYES

In middle school Seth complained about headaches. By now I understood that visual acuity and visual constancy are paramount for learning, and that any visual impairment interferes with development.

In *Children with Cerebral Palsy: A Parents' Guide*, I read there are very common vision problems among children with cerebral palsy. The symptoms are indicative of underlying disorders including sensory delays that affect balance and body awareness, trouble discerning backgrounds from foregrounds, and so on.

Autistic people often use visual information inefficiently. They have problems coordinating their central and peripheral vision.

I consulted Dr. Richard Kavner, a vision specialist and behavioral optometrist. His specialty is "vision training." Dr. Kavner believes that vision skills can be improved through exercise and nutrition geared to the eyes.

In his book, *Total Vision*, Dr. Kavner defines behavioral optometry as the combined knowledge of psychology, neurology, biology, child development, and other related fields. He writes that our eyes are receptors of the brain.

The eye is not just a camera, but a part of the entire visual apparatus, which begins and ends at the back of the brain. The eyes take in the data and channel it along neural impulses to the cortex, where the central control makes sense out of the information.

Case studies demonstrate that enhancing or expanding vision changes personality and behavior. This theory melded perfectly with the information I was getting from training in Feldenkrais teachings, studying Glenn Doman, and my increasing interest in somatics not to mention my Iyengar practice that remains at the center of my life.

When vision changes, so does personality and behavior. This is why Iyengar always gives instruction about where to put the eyes in every pose. (And specific instructions about how to close them.) As Dr. Kavner explains, our eyes are active seekers of the essence of life, constantly searching, scanning, and selecting from the environment.

The eye is a living organ that is always in communication with other vital centers of the body. What we think and how we feel are constant companions of the images we pay attention to.

FLEXYX/BIOFEEDBACK NEURODEVELOPMENTAL THERAPY

When Seth was a teenager, I heard about a treatment known as Flexyx. It was described as a holistic, synergistic approach to biofeedback. I thought maybe Flexyx would be good for someone with cerebral palsy. I was right. And it appears to be excellent for many, many brain injuries, although the research is not yet complete.

Since 1990, Len Ochs, Ph.D., has been developing a form of EEG Biofeedback, which utilizes both light and electromagnetic stimulation to reduce the brainwave dysregulation underlying many neurological, psychological and physical conditions. His method is called the Flexyx Neurotherapy System.

We were open to whatever would help Seth and were excited

to learn of the availability of this program in New York City. After reading the literature and meeting with Dr. Steven Larsen at Stone Mountain Counseling Center, we were convinced we should try Flexyx. Going for this is an example of what it means to take one experience into another.

In October 1998 Seth began the course of treatments, and there were immediate observable results. He was a sophomore in high school and suffered from stress. There was so much work, and his stamina once again became an issue. He experienced difficulty sleeping and the combination of physical exhaustion and sleep deprivation caused more spasticity and involuntary movement and even very dramatic mood swings. He frequently lost his temper, which was something new.

We were concerned that he would not be able to sustain his focus and stamina. He wanted to go to a top college, and so he needed to get good grades and be calm and clear for the required testing. He put a lot of pressure on himself. From the very beginning of his Flexyx therapy, he became calmer and slept more easily. His speech was clearer and his gross and fine motor skills seemed smoother. His work in school improved. A general sense of optimism prevailed. The word I used as soon as I saw Seth after his first treatment was "grounded". He seemed to have his feet on the ground with new attitude. I was reminded of a first grade boy I saw swinging from a gate after school on the day after his first treatment with Frymann.

GROWING

When Seth was seven he got scary sick. We did everything we could for him and took him to the doctor, but they found nothing especially wrong as far as a cold or infection. For those few days we were very frightened. The doctors discouraged us from taking him to the emergency room. We were ready to do so in any case when Seth began to improve.

Up until then Seth's one absolute personal characteristic was his lack of stamina. He was intelligent, enthusiastic, sociable, irascible, but he fatigued rapidly. He always required twelve hours of sleep every night.

Suddenly, that was no longer the case. Not only was he more energetic than ever before, he was vigorous. He no longer slept as much. He stopped complaining about being tired.

When Dr. Frymann examined Seth she told us he had "shed an old skin." She remarked that children often experience an extreme malady prior to a significant neurological and/or physiological and/or emotional transformation.

Each child—with or without disabilities—may experience a form of "growing pains" prior to developmental milestones. For example, a child can get cranky and fitful just before learning to walk independently. Because of Seth's cerebral palsy, this illness was more drastic and upsetting, but in some ways it affirmed his "normalcy."

HEARING

Deafness is the most common disability present at birth. However, a deaf newborn looks and acts like any other baby.

Often allopathic physicians do not detect deafness until a child is two or three. Such delays can permanently impair a child's ability to learn to speak intelligibly and can result in long lasting, social, emotional and academic difficulties.

Dr. Frymann often discussed hearing loss. She taught that "…the ear is not something sitting out in space. The ear is part of the total mechanism of the body." It is encased in the temporal bone and because of the trauma or injury at birth the rhythm of the temporal bone is restricted.

As a result, it is common for little children to get frequent ear infections. It is not unusual to hear mothers admit that their child has had ear infections over and over again. In fact today ear infections have reached epic proportions and even after long courses of antibiotics children do not get well.

LEARNING

In the Feldenkrais trainings the importance of timing and comfort were continually emphasized. I recognized that an unpleasant learning experience can hamper the entire learning process.

Feldenkrais said, "learning involves an improvement of the brain function itself. To facilitate learning it is necessary to divorce the aim to be achieved from the learning process itself.

"The process is the important thing and should be aimless to the adult learner just as is learning to the baby. The baby is not held to any timetable, nor is there any need to rely on force."

These were very important concepts for me to keep in mind as I thought about Seth's progress. And it strongly relates to my Iyengar yoga practice.

PSYCHOTHERAPY

We engaged a psychologist to test Seth and help us pinpoint weaknesses along his learning curve. During a difficult time when Seth was in the first grade, we also submitted him to the tests at the Board of Education.

In addition to the testing, our psychologist helped us with strategies for dealing with Seth in stressful situations. He helped us sort out how to wake Seth in the morning, especially after a night when he was waking frequently; he helped us ameliorate the obvious understandable fact that when he was in the first grade Seth did not want to go to school (who could blame him?). Seth was late for school every day.

The doctor made suggestions to the school, and we asked them to cooperate in strategies to deal with Seth's lateness. The doctor's involvement legitimized our requests at school. He helped us to be consistent.

We initiated systems for rule making, which included getting Seth's agreement. We began to recognize how much Seth was used to having his own way.

Around this time Jay and I met with Dr. Frymann. The doctor told us that Seth was struggling for control in his life and struggling with her, too. (This pattern was already familiar from our days with Anat and Charles.)

She wanted us to clearly establish the lines of acceptable behavior for him. She told us to constantly orient him to solutions rather than problems. Dr. Frymann said a child needs time to unwind and to fantasize through play, song, creative occupations, time every day just to be at peace. We became acutely aware of the demands Seth faced to do the 'work' of school, go to therapy and function. Down time was as important as could be and I began to be sure he had it.

SPEECH

Dr. Frymann always encouraged me to think of Seth's speech and articulation difficulties as mainly a problem of proper breathing. After all my years of study with Carola Speads and all I saw from working on Seth myself I agreed. I put effort into finding someone who would work with Seth like this. Thankfully, I was already seriously studying and practicing Iyengar Yoga that I met a fellow student who was working with a breath coach, Carl Stough, known as "Dr. Breath."

Carl Stough acquired his sobriquet during the Olympics in Mexico City when he prepared the United States Olympic track team. Mexico City's high altitude alters breathing, making more demands on a runner's lung power. Stough came to the rescue, coaching the team in breathing techniques that helped them win many gold medals. Opera singers, trumpeters, pop vocalists, musicians, body workers, many others were students of Carl Stough. His students also included people suffering from serious emphysema.

So much of the work Carl Stough did with Seth related to what I learned in Carola's studio years earlier. The work was centered in the breath. The lessons revitalized Seth, changed his carriage, his voice, and his alignment.

Seth saw Dr. Stough once a week for years. I never heard him complain once about going. It is not easy for a young boy and then an adolescent young man to do this kind of work consistently and comprehend its value. What made it possible for Seth was two-fold: we were very supportive and made it available and it was a place where he experienced great revitalization and renewal. (Plus he ran into a lot of celebrities!)

Seth continued using vocal coaches after Stough died. Through my connections in the theater world I drew on referrals for professionals who had studied with Kristin Linklater and others. (Kristin Linklater is a Scottish vocal coach, dialect coach, acting teacher, actor, theatre director, and author. She is currently Head of Acting in the Theatre Arts Division of Columbia University.)

Think *The King's Speech*!

APPENDIX (A-Z)

This Appendix provides detailed descriptions of therapies and methodologies referenced in the book including links for further exploration.

BIOFEEDBACK

Biofeedback is a treatment technique in which people are trained to improve their health by using signals from their own bodies. By responding to these signals patients learn to self-regulate body and mind function. Physical therapists use biofeedback to help stroke victims regain movement in paralyzed muscles. Psychologists use it to help tense and anxious clients learn to relax.

Specialists in many different fields use biofeedback to help their patients cope with pain. Biofeedback makes use of electronic monitoring of a normally automatic bodily function in order to train someone to acquire voluntary control of that function. Biofeedback as a mind-body method is one of the most widely accepted modalities of the complementary family of interventions.

With biofeedback, you are often connected to electrical sensors that help you receive information (feedback) about your body (bio). This feedback helps you focus on making subtle changes in your body, such as relaxing certain muscles, to achieve the results you want, like reducing pain. In essence, biofeedback gives you the power to use your thoughts to control your body, often to improve a health condition or physical performance.

There are a wide range and different methods of biofeedback. A therapist might use several different biofeedback methods in combination. Determining the method that's right for you depends on your health problems and goals. Biofeedback methods include brainwave, breathing, EEG, virtual reality and other non-cognitive monitoring and stimulation experiments too numerous to detail within the scope of this Appendix.

You can receive biofeedback training in physical therapy clinics, medical centers and hospitals with various devices. A growing number of biofeedback devices and programs are also being marketed for home use, including interactive computer or mobile device programs, wearable devices like headbands, computer graphics for home use on multiple electronic plat-forms. Many biofeedback devices marketed for home use are not regulated by the Food and Drug Administration. Before trying biofeedback therapy at home, discuss the different types of devices with your doctor to find the best fit.

See The Association for Applied Psychophysiology and Biofeedback (http://www.aapb.org/)

CRANIAL OSTEOPATHY

Cranial osteopathy is a specialized form of osteopathic medicine that follows the teachings of Dr. William Sutherland. Osteopaths who have studied and specialized in this system maintain that because of the linkage in the system of fascial tissue and the vertebral column through the sacrum, palpation of the skull and sacrum can pick up rhythmic pulsation distinct from the respiratory rhythm or the heartbeat and pulse of the blood. This pulsation is the reverberation of the cerebrospinal fluid, which bathes both the brain and the spinal column.

Restrictions that result from injury or inflexibility in the spine and cranium can cause abnormal motion in the craniosacral system. This abnormal motion leads to stresses that can contribute to poor health, especially in the brain and spinal cord.

The purpose of craniosacral therapy is to enhance the functioning of this system. The relationship of one cranial bone to the other is normalized, and the cerebrospinal fluid pressure is adjusted. As a result, the whole physiology of the central nervous system functions more efficiently.

Common conditions such as earaches, sinus congestion, vomiting, irritability, and hyperactivity have been successfully treated using only craniosacral therapy. Osteopathic physicians who are trained in cranial osteopathy use their techniques to identify all kinds of disturbed patterns of movement, to diagnose and treat many disorders in a gentle, noninvasive way, and the effects of this treatment can be very far reaching.

In his book, *New Way to Health: a Guide to Osteopathy,* Stephen Sandler, D.O., describes the cranial osteopath as a highly trained physician who uses refined hands-on techniques to detect and treat subtle disturbances in motion patterns of the skull, which are often symptomatic of certain disorders.

Sandler describes how osteopaths who have studied and specialized in cranial work maintain that palpation on the skull and sacrum picks up a rhythmic pulsation distinct from the respiratory rhythm or the heartbeat and pulse of the blood. This pulsation is the reverberation of the cerebrospinal fluid, which bathes both the brain and the spinal column.

Cranial osteopaths explain that the brain is suspended inside the skull by sheets of tissue known as the meninges. These meninges extend all the way down the vertebral column to the sacrum. This linkage connects the movement of the skull bones and the movement of the pelvis. Cranial work inclines to balance the rhythmical forces at work in the body by gently guiding and releasing the tensions within the reciprocal tension of these tissues.

Children in particular respond well to the gentle approach of this treatment. It is especially helpful in assisting children to attain full recovery after common childhood illnesses, but also after such episodes as falls or traumatic birthtic birth" s.

Some of the most successful craniosacral treatments are performed on newborns and infants. At this stage the cranial bones are primarily cartilage and the membranes are growing and changing very rapidly so the child is very responsive to the gentle corrections of the therapist's fingers.

*Cranial osteopaths are trained medical doctors. Dr. John Upledger, an osteopath trained craniosacral practitioners who may not have training in anatomy or physiology, and while the therapy is harmless in itself, medical doctors fear that these practitioners may fail to recognize serious medical conditions. Upledger, who was an osteopath at Michigan State University, incorporated some of the techniques from cranial osteopathy—distinguishing it from cranial osteopathy in being "soft tissued," "fluid oriented," and "membrane oriented," rather than "bone oriented."

See Anne Woodham and Dr. David Peters's book, *The Encyclopedia of Healing Therapies.*

See The Cranial Academy (http://cranialacademy.org/)

ERICKSON HYPNOTHERAPY

Milton H. Erickson was an American psychiatrist and psychologist specializing in medical hypnosis and family therapy and was acknowledged as the foremost authority on hypnotherapy and brief strategic psychotherapy. Many Feldenkrais practitioners subscribe closely to the work of Milton Erickson.

Erickson surmounted enormous health problems throughout his adult life. Confined to a wheelchair, color deficient, practically quadriplegic, he retrained himself in everything. And he believed that it was these very challenges that were the best teachers about human behavior and potentials.

Both Feldenkrais and Erickson believed that the widening of awareness through movement occurs unconsciously. They believed learning happens to a large degree through the unconscious functioning of the nervous system. It is the nervous system that has the life experience of the individual available to it, as well as the biological wisdom gained through the process of evolution. The learning process is the important thing; it must be aimless.

Erickson taught that the power to change is something that lies dormant within the individual and needs only to be reawakened. He was a proponent of the idea that therapy is anything that changes the habitual pattern of behavior.

Erickson believed that our unconscious mind knows more than we do. The conscious mind is our state of immediate awareness. The unconscious mind is made up of all our learning over a lifetime, much of which has been forgotten by the conscious mind but nonetheless serves us in our automatic functioning. In other words, our brain cells are so specialized that we have literally a brain cell for every item of knowledge, and they are all connected. *See* https://www.erickson-foundation.org/biography/

FELDENKRAIS

Moshe Feldenkrais was a Russian-born (1904) Israeli scientist with a black belt in Judo, (the first European to hold the black belt). He was an electrical and mechanical engineer, and a mathematician. He also worked as a researcher on the French atomic bomb program.

In the 1940's Feldenkrais developed a method to explore

body awareness, improve flexibility and confidence and enhance well-being. He believed that we could break age-old self-destructive patterns of movement, influence the brain to change hurtful body movements, and improve quality of life and functioning through body movement awareness and skill. He believed that the emotional and nervous systems can be "taught" to heal the physical person. This process is known as "sensory reeducation."

These ends are accomplished with special exercises that reorganize and stimulate parts of the brain and initiate new learning. Students learn from their own sensorimotor experience by using the process of "childhood organic learning." Learning comes from doing and is greatly dependent on the unconscious functioning of the nervous system. Learning itself is seen as a powerful therapeutic and self-actualizing force.

The Feldenkrais method questioned some very basic and established premises that had guided physical rehabilitation practices for many decades. The method is an educational system, not a therapeutic system. The exercises are designed to improve function rather than correct it. Learning is engendered not necessarily through moving, but through awareness of the process of moving.

There are two aspects to the learning:

One phase is known as *Functional Integration*. It is accomplished by a one-on-one relationship between the therapist and the student to achieve increased mobility and control. This manipulative treatment is slow, gentle, and painless.

The other aspect to the learning, taught in groups, is called *Awareness through Movement (ATM)*. ATM is a learning process that makes self-direction easier.

In both methods the student *learns to learn* how to attend to his or her particular movements with greater awareness. The student learns to refine the details of his or her actions.

See http://www.feldenkrais.com/whatis and http://feldenk-rais-method.org

FLEXYX NEUROFEEDBACK

Trauma of any kind (physical, infectious, toxic or emotional) causes brain waves to become fixated or "stuck" in a pattern of predominantly slow brainwave activity called "EEG slowing." Researchers believe EEG slowing is the way in which the brain protects itself from seizures and stimulation overload by releasing neurochemicals that protect it from any further danger. Unfortunately, this protective reaction also interferes with efficient neurological communications and causes the person to lose functional abilities in the areas of energy regulation, cognitive processing and mood modulation.

Dr. Len Ochs discovered that brains considered physically damaged beyond repair could be partially or totally rehabilitated, sometimes years after the initial injury, by treatment with this method. Research with light and sound stimulation had already proved useful in helping children with autism and learning disabilities. Dr. Ochs was asked to design a system that combined both EEG biofeedback and Light/Sound technology and therapy based on this research.

Basically, the Flexyx Neurofeedback System (FNS) is an advanced form of EEG biofeedback, which uses imperceptible light (from tiny LEDs) or infinitesimally weak electromagnetic pulses as the feedback signal. The system, in general, operates by monitoring patient's' brainwaves.

People sit in a chair, eyes closed, wearing dark glasses that have a set of tiny lights mounted in the lenses. They are exposed to various amounts of the stimulation depending on their levels of sensitivity and responsiveness. With the help of sophisticated computer technology, the patient's dominant, or strongest, frequency brainwave is monitored and used to control the frequency rate at which the stimulation is delivered.

The length of the session and intensity of the stimulation are carefully adjusted to balance clinical effectiveness and patient comfort. The lights are programmed to pulsate at a slightly different frequency rate from the momentary dominant frequency in the patient's brain.

The basic premise is to interrupt the brain's rigid defensive pattern and stimulate it to develop a wider and more flexible range of responsiveness on the bioelectrical and neurochemical level. These brainwave changes eventually translate into a greater 'flexibility' both neurologically and behaviorally.

Use of Flexyx therapy has resulted in rather significant alleviation of symptoms in conditions as varied as attention deficit disorder and post-traumatic stress to stroke and spinal cord injury, depression, headache, speech and fine motor skill and other problems.

See http://www.site.ochslabs.com/ and

Stone Mountain Counseling Center

HOMEOPATHY

As explained in the *Family Guide to Natural Medicine,* homeopathy dates formally from the year 1810 and the publication of Samuel Hahnemann's *Organon of Medicine.*

Hahnemann, a German physician and chemist deplored most popular medical procedures as "heroic," preferring to treat the whole patient instead of the disease. Homeopaths believe that illness is not localized in one organ, but instead involves the entire person, both body and mind. Homeopathy is based on two major principles, the Law of Similars and the Law of Infinitesimals.

Simply put, the Law of Similars states, "Like cures like." A substance that produces a certain set of symptoms in a healthy person has the power to cure a sick person manifesting those same symptoms.

The Law of Infinitesimals states that the smaller the dose of a remedy, when properly diluted, the more effective it will be in stimulating the body's vital forces to react against disease. A third principle, the Law of Chronic Disease, states that when disease persists despite treatment, it is the result of one or more conditions that affect many people and have been driven deep inside the body by earlier allopathic therapy.

See https://nccih.nih.gov/health/homeopathy

IYENGAR YOGA

Iyengar Yoga, named after and developed by B. K. S. Iyengar, is a form of Hatha Yoga that emphasizes detail, precision and alignment in the performance of posture (*asana*) and breath control (*pranayama*). The development of strength, mobility and stability is gained through the *asanas* and the practice of *pranayama*.

As Mr. Iyengar taught: yoga means union, the union of the individual soul with the universal spirit. Yoga is a discipline that removes all dualities and divisions. It integrates body with breath, breath with mind, mind with intelligence and intelligence with the Soul. "Yoga is both an evolutive path (onward journey) and involutive path (inward journey) in the quest of the soul." Yoga requires tremendous effort, perseverance and patience.

Iyengar Yoga often makes use of props, such as belts, blocks, and blankets, as aids in performing asanas (postures). The props enable students to perform the asanas correctly, minimizing the risk of injury or strain, and making the postures accessible to both young and old.

Iyengar yoga is known to be highly effective in relieving and/ or curing chronic ailments from skeleto/muscular divergences, circulatory problems, digestive and respiratory disorders. People who are HIV positive are finding improvement in the quality of their lives after Iyengar yoga. There are special classes for such people in the USA and France. There are also special classes to treat addiction as well as classes for veterans, breast cancer survivors and amputees

Iyengar yoga is a complete approach to physical, mental, emotional, and spiritual transformation, bringing physical health, vitality, mental clarity, wisdom, and emotional serenity. As Mr. Iyengar said, the end of discipline is the beginning of freedom. Mary Dunn described Mr. Iyengar brilliantly when she wrote on the occasion of Mr. Iyengar's 70th birthday, "....Mr. Iyengar has the brain of a scientist, the mind of an artist, and the soul of a seer."

See https://iynaus.org/iyengar-yoga

NDT: "meurodevelopmental" method of physical therapy/the bobath method

This method is the one most commonly used for infants and children with cerebral palsy in the United States. Karl and Berta Bobath, a husband and wife introduced it in the 1950s from England, and it is considered very mainstream.

The NDT approach helps prepare the child's posture and movement to permit the development of "functional skills" or those skills needed for feeding, dressing, and bathing, i.e. the skills that are basic to living independently.

Treatment focuses on encouraging the child to use normal rather than abnormal movement patterns and on preventing deformities or muscle patterns that make developing movement skills.

See

http://www.bobath.org.uk/for-commissioners/bobath-therapy/

For neurodevelopmental therapy, the following site and book are helpfl: https://www.ndta.org/whatisndt.php and *Bobath Concept: Theory and Clinical Practice in Neurological Rehabilitation*

OSTEOPATHY

Osteopathy is the oldest bona fide medical healing art and osteopathy is a holistic approach to diagnosis and treatment. Osteopaths are primary-care physicians, licensed to practice medicine, perform surgery, and dispense drugs. D.O.s are trained to be doctors first, and specialists second. Doctors of osteopathy (D.O.s) and M.D.s (allopathic physicians) are the only two types of complete physicians. Doctors of osteopathy practice in all branches of medicine and surgery, from psychiatry to obstetrics, from geriatrics to emergency medicine. Osteopathy originated in the United States in the late 19th century. Now established alongside conventional medicine in North America and practiced throughout Europe, and Australasia, osteopathy is one of the most respected and widely used complementary therapies. Osteopathy is a *manual examination and treatment method* of the integrated musculoskeletal, visceral system and craniosacral systems. A certified osteopath examines and manually treats the mobility of all these systems and looks for limitations in mobility that could be linked to the patient's complaint.

Osteopaths believe that the manipulation of bones, the *palpation* of tissue, and the use of osteopathic manipulative therapy (OMT) re-establish the structural integrity of the body, leading to the free flow of blood. The musculoskeletal system is used as the basic approach to the patient but osteopath's range of actions includes all body systems.

While MD's (allopathic physicians) think of the body as a number of discrete systems, doctors of osteopathy (D.O.'s) view the body as an interrelated whole, with each system and organ in constant contact with the other and others. They believe that the body's structure plays a critical role in its ability to function.

Osteopaths use their eyes and a battery of manual techniques to identify structural problems. They focus on the neuromusculoskeletal system (the bones, muscles, tendons, tissues, nerves, spinal column, and brain) and work to support the body's natural tendency toward health and self-healing.

Osteopaths are not chiropractors. Chiropractors are not physicians and have not had the training of an osteopath and their objectives are limited to alignment and symmetry. More importantly, for osteopaths the act of manipulation is more than a physical act. The osteopath is trained to know what the norm should be and recognizes—without judgement—the deviations. Osteopaths resonate through the structure of the body and believe you can "listen to your hands." (Frymann)

Function and integration is the goal of osteopathy. The intention in osteopathy is to help life come into balance in the way it intends. The theory is that all bodies are in process; they are not static. This view of process is also essential to the somatic vision.

The manipulative techniques osteopaths use are designed to improve circulation and stimulate the immune system fostering change in a preventative way, helping us become less susceptible to toxic stimulants in the environment.

Osteopathic manipulative therapy (OMT) recognizes that there is a systematic integrity in each individual, that there is a self-balancing and self-adjusting ability in the human species. Osteopathy accounts for the entire function of the body, bones being considered the foundation for the body's structure and therefore its function.

Osteopathy can be especially valuable in helping to diagnose and treat developmental problems in children. Dr. Frymann said that only ten percent of children have normal body structure. Ten percent of children have distortion that is visible to the naked eye. Eighty percent of children's structural distortions are not visible. She said eighty percent of children with learning problems have suffered difficult births.

Osteopaths use their hands diagnostically, perceptually, and therapeutically. The founder of osteopathy was an M.D. surgeon, Dr. Andrew Taylor Still, who trained physicians to use their hands for healing along with simple and natural remedies – diet, rest, meditation, prayer.

See http://doctorsthatdo.org/ and http://www.osteopathie.eu/en

PLASTICITY

A young child's nervous system is still forming and this plasticity in a child's central nervous system gives it an ability to recover completely or partially after an insult to the brain. For this reason the brains of very young children have a greater capacity to repair themselves than do adult brains. A child's central nervous system produces many more brain cells and connections than are eventually used for complex motor tasks. As a result as long as a child's nervous system has not yet matured, there is still a chance that the child can make at least a partial recovery from early movement problems.

The brains of infants and young children repair themselves more frequently than do those of older children (thus the importance of early intervention).

As the nervous system organizes over time, motor abilities and other abilities are affected differently. If a brain injury occurs early, the undamaged areas of a child's brain can often take over some of the functions of the damaged areas.

SOMATICS

Somatics refers to practices in the field of movement studies that emphasize internal physical perception. The term is used in movement therapy to signify an approach based on the *soma*, or "the body as perceived from within,"[1] and in dance as an antonym for "performative techniques"—such as ballet or modern dance—that emphasize the external observation of movement by an audience. Somatic techniques may be used in bodywork, psychotherapy, dance, or spiritual practices.

The first time I read about Somatics was in the work of Thomas Hanna, who writes extensively about how humans function best. Mr. Hanna was the editor of the magazine *Somatics* and was the author of several books and the director of the Novato Institute for Somatic Research and Training in California.

See http://hannasomatics.com/index.php, http://somaticsed.com/ and http:/somaticstudies.com/ruella-frank/

SUGGESTED READING
Books to further inform your journey.

A Leg to Stand On by Oliver Sacks
The Brain that Changes Itself by Norman Doidge
The Brain's Way of Healing: Remarkable Discoveries and Recoveries from the Frontiers of Neuroplasticity by Norman Doidge
The Busy Person's Guide to Easier Movement by Frank Wildman
The Care of the Soul by Thomas Moore
The Dancing Wu Li Masters by Gary Zukav
Discipline: The Brazelton Way by Joshua D. Sparrow
From My Hands and Heart: Achieving Health and Balance by Kate Mackinnon
Health and Healing: Understanding Conventional and Alternative Medicine by Andrew Weill
How the Brain Heals Itself (with a chapter on Feldenkrais) by Norman Doidge
In a Different Key by John Donvan and Caren Zucker
Infants and Mothers: Differences in Development by T. Berry Brazleton
Joy: The Surrender to the Body by Alexander Lowen
Kids Beyond Limits: The Anat Baniel Method for Awakening the Brain by Anat Baniel

Life Animated: for Heroes and Sidekicks by Ron Suskind
Light on Life by B.K.S. Iyengar
Love that Boy by Ron Fournier
The Man Who Mistook His Wife for a Hat by Oliver Sacks
Move into Life: Neuromovement for Lifelong Vitality by Anat Baniel
On Becoming a Family by T. Berry Brazleton
Philosophy of Osteopathy by Andrew Still
Quantum Healing by Deepak Chopra
The Seat of the Soul by Gary Zukav
*Somatics: Reawakening the Mind's Control of Movement, Flexibility
    and Health* by Thomas Hanna
Space, Time, and Medicine by Larry Dossey
Tao of Physics by Fritjof Capra
Touchpoints: Birth to Three by T. Berry Brazelton
*Touchpoints: Three to Six (Your Child's Emotional and Behavioral
    Development)* by T. Berry Brazelton
Train Go Sorry, Leah Coen Hager
Waking: A Memoir of Trauma and Transcendence by Matthew Sanford
The World According to Mister Rogers by Fred Rogers
Yoga the Iyengar Way by Mira Mehta
Yoga: the Path to Holistic Health by BKS Iyengar

GLOSSARY

These definitions are from multiple sources as well as my personal knowledge and experience. Pursue links to the Appendix and Resource Guide for further exploration.

accommodation (in IEP): a change to a task that enables a child to complete it.

acupuncture: a natural and holistic Chinese therapy that inserts needles into pressure points.

adaptive physical education: physical education that has been adapted or modified so that it is as appropriate for the person with a disability as it is for a person without a disability.

Alexander technique: a method developed to move mindfully through life and remove tension and pain.

alloparent: one who is not the biological parent and performs the role of parent.

allopathic: the treatment of disease by conventional means, i.e., with drugs having opposite effects to the symptoms.

amniocentesis: a prenatal test performed by removing amniotic fluid from the uterus.

auditory blending: the ability to perceive individual sounds (especially parts of words) as parts of a whole, in particular to understand words.

autism: a general or "umbrella" term used to describe a group of complex disorders that affect brain development. According to autism.org, it is defined as "...a lifelong, developmental disability that affects how a person communicates with and relates to other people, and how they experience the world around them."

Ayurvedic medicine: Considered by many scholars to be the oldest healing science, Ayurveda is a holistic approach to health designed to help people live long, healthy, balanced lives (*https://nccih.nih.gov/health/ ayurveda*).

behavioral optometry/optometrist: a system of eye care that emphasizes visual training as a way to improve the way a patient uses his or her eyes. Behavioral optometrists attempt to train the patient to see better across a range of different circumstances rather than just prescribing lenses.

biofeedback: a technique that trains people to improve their health by controlling certain controlling certain bodily processes that normally happen involuntarily, such as heart rate, blood pressure, muscle tension, and skin temperature. *See Appendix.*

Bobath method: a neurodevelopmental (also known as NDT) approach for assessment and treatment of individuals with cerebral palsy and other allied neurological conditions. *See Appendix.*

cerebral palsy: a neurological disorder caused by a non-progressive brain injury or malformation that occurs while a child's brain is under development, affecting body movement and muscle coordination. Though Cerebral Palsy can be defined, having cerebral palsy does not define the person who has the condition.

child study team: a multidisciplinary group of professionals typically employed by the board of education to provide parents and teachers with a variety of learning related services.

cranial osteopathy: a variety of osteopathic manipulative therapies that stimulate healing using gentle hand pressure to manipulate the skeleton and connective tissues, especially the skull. *See Appendix.*

cranial-sacral therapy: a holistic healing practice that uses very light touching to balance the craniosacral system in the body, which includes the bones, nerves, fluids, and connective tissues of the cranium and spinal area. (https://www.craniosacraltherapy.org)

developmental disability: a severe, chronic disability that originates at birth or during childhood, is expected to continue indefinitely, and substantially restricts the individual's functioning in several major life activities. (http://www.ddrcco.com/resources-and-training/definition-of-developmental-disability.php)

early intervention: a system of services that helps babies and toddlers with developmental delays or disabilities, focusing on helping these babies and toddlers learn the basic and brand-new skills that typically develop during the first three years of life (crawling, walking, learning, problem-solving, talking, playing, eating, etc.).(http://www.parentcenterhub.org/repository/ei-overview/)

FAPE (Free Appropriate Public Education): the Individuals with Disabilities Education Act says that each child who has a disability and needs special education and related services will receive a *free and appropriate public education.*

Feldenkrais: named for Moshe Feldenkrais, this is a method to explore body awareness, improve flexibility and enhance well-being. *See Appendix.*

Flexyx: a process that restores flexibility to the nervous system, and hence revitalizes functioning. *See Appendix.*

genetic counseling: Genetic counseling is the process of evaluating family history and medical records through genetic tests—including the evaluation of the results—and helping parents understand and reach decisions about what to do next.

homeopathy: a medical science based on the principle that any substance that can produce symptoms in a healthy person can cure similar symptoms in a person who is sick. *See Appendix.*

IDEA: the Individuals with Disabilities Education Act; a federal law that outlines rights and regulations for students with disabilities in the United States who require special education.

IEP: Individualized Education Program; an important legal document for children who receive special education service that spells out the child's learning needs, the services the school will provide, and how progress will be measured.

Local education agency (LEA): commonly-used synonym for a school district, an entity that operates local public primary and secondary schools in the US.

LRE: Least Restrictive Environment; part of the IDEA that states that children who receive special education should learn in the least restrictive environment, meaning they should spend as much time as possible with their peers who do not receive special education.

mainstreaming: when a school puts children with special needs into classrooms with their peers who have no disabilities.

meconium: the first fecal excretion of a newborn child.

multiple sclerosis (MS): an unpredictable, often disabling disease of the central nervous system that disrupts the flow of information within the brain, and between the brain and body

Myers-Briggs: a widely-used personality inventory, or test, employed in vocational, educational, and psychotherapy settings to evaluate personality type in adolescents and adults age 14 and older.

neural impulse: an electrical discharge that travels along a nerve fiber.

NDT (Neurodevelopmental Therapy): a therapeutic approach to the assessment and management dysfunction in people with neurological impairments. The ultimate goal of treatment and management is to maximize the person's functional ability. *See Appendix.*

NICU (Neonatal Intensive Care Unit): a special area of the hospital for newborn babies who require intensive medical attention.

occipital artery: a branch of the external carotid, the occipital artery begins in the neck and runs to the back of the head transporting oxygenated blood to many regions throughout the body.

occupational therapy: a therapy to help people do the things they want and need to do through the therapeutic use of daily activities (occupations).

orthotic: A support, brace, or splint used to support, align, prevent, or correct the function of movable parts of the body.

osteopathy: a form of drug-free non-invasive manual medicine that focuses on total body health. Its aim is to positively affect the body's nervous, circulatory, and lymphatic systems by treating and strengthening the musculoskeletal framework, which includes the joints, muscles and spine. *See Appendix.*

palpation: the act of feeling with the hand; the application of the fingers with light pressure to the surface of the body for the purpose of determining the condition of the parts beneath in physical diagnosis.

pediatric physical therapist: one who treats and examines children from birth to age 18 who have problems moving and performing other physical activities. Pediatric physical therapists help treat problems like injuries, pre-existing conditions, and problems caused by illnesses or diseases.

pediatric neurology: a specialized branch of medicine that deals with the diagnosis and management of neurological conditions in infants, children and adolescents.

pediatric orthopedist: evaluates and treats bone, joint, or muscle problems in children who are still growing.

pediatric podiatry: the specialized care and treatment of disorders and conditions of children's feet.

plasticity: the brain's ability to change at any age. *See Appendix.*

prodromal labor: a type of labor that happens prior to the onset of full active labor. Often considered a type of "false labor" (a misnomer). The contractions are real but they start and stop.

Public Law 94: Education for All Handicapped Children Act, signed into law in 1975.

RTI (Response to Intervention): a system of learning mostly applied to students with special needs due to their difficulty when it comes to learning. Its main objective is to identify the weakness in a child and develop strategies to enable the child learn effectively, regardless of how long it takes.

sacrum: the large, triangular bone at the base of the spinal column. *See cranial-sacral therapy.*

sensorimotor learning: the improvement, through practice, in the performance of sensory-guided motor behavior.

Somatics: a form of neuromuscular (mind-body training) movement re-education that goes directly to the root cause of most chronic muscular pain: the brain and the way in which it senses and organizes the muscles and movement. *See Appendix*

stress test: a test to gather information about how your heart works during physical activity. Because exercise makes your heart pump harder and faster than usual, an exercise stress test can reveal problems within your heart that might not be noticeable otherwise.

BIBLIOGRAPHY

Baniel, Anat. *Kids beyond Limits: the Anat Baniel Method for Awakening the Brain and Transforming the Life of Your Child with Special Needs.* New York, NY, Perigee Trade, 2012.

Baniel, Anat. *Move into Life: NeuroMovement for Lifelong Vitality.* San Rafael, CA, Crowning Beauty, 2015.

Baskin, Amy. "How to Keep Your Relationship Strong While Parenting a Special Needs Child." *Today's Parent*, Rogers Digital Media, 18 June 2013, www.todaysparent.com/family/parenting/how-to-keep-your-relationship-strong-while-parenting-a-special-needs-child/.

Bateson, Gregory. *Mind and Nature: a Necessary Unity.* Toronto, Bantam Books, 1980.

Batshaw, Mark et al. *Children with Disabilities, Seventh Edition.* Newburyport, Brookes Publishing, 2014.

Batshaw, Mark L. *When Your Child Has a Disability: the Complete Sourcebook of Daily and Medical Care.* Baltimore, MD, Paul H. Brookes Publishing Co., 2001.

Boston Women's Health Book Collective. *Ourselves and Our Children: a Book by and for Parents*. New York, Random House, 1978.

Brazelton, T. Berry, and Joshua D. Sparrow. *Discipline: the Brazelton Way*. Cambridge, MA, Perseus Publishers, 2003.

Brazelton, T. Berry. *On Becoming a Family: the Growth of Attachment*. New York, Delacorte Press/Seymour Lawrence, 1981.

Brazelton, T. Berry, and Joshua D. Sparrow. *Touchpoints Three to Six: Your Child's Emotional and Behavioral Development*. Cambridge, MA, Perseus Publishers, 2001.

Buck, Pearl S. *The Child Who Never Grew*. New York, J. Day Co., 1950.

Burgess, Rick, Bubba Bussey, and Martha Bolton. *Rick and Bubba's Guide to the Almost Nearly Perfect Marriage*. Nashville, TN, Thomas Nelson, 2009.

Capra, Fritjof. *The Tao of Physics: an Exploration of the Parallels between Modern Physics and Eastern Mysticism*. Berkeley, Shambhala, 1975.

Cassileth, Barrie R. *The Alternative Medicine Handbook, The Complete Reference Guide to Alternative and Complementary Therapies*. 1st ed., New York, W. W. Norton & Company, 1998.

Chanchani, Swati, and Rajiv Chanchani. *Yoga for Children: a Complete Illustrated Guide to Yoga: Including a Manual for Parents and Teachers*. New Delhi, UBS Publishers' Distributors Ltd., 1995.

Chodron, Pema. *When Things Fall Apart: Heart Advice for Difficult Times*. Boston, Shambhala, 1997.

Cohen, Sherry Suib. *The Magic of Touch*. New York, Harper & Row, 1987.

Cohen, Leah Hager. *Train Go Sorry: Inside a Deaf World*. Boston, Houghton Mifflin, 1994.

Criswell, Eleanor. *How Yoga Works: an Introduction to Somatic Yoga*. Novato, CA, Freeperson Press, 1987.

Doman, Glenn J. *What to Do about Your Brain-Injured Child: or Your Brain-Damaged, Mentally Retarded, Mentally Deficient, Cerebral-Palsied, Epileptic, Autistic, Athetoid, Hyperactive, Attention Deficit Disordered, Developmentally Delayed, down's Child*. Garden City Park, NY, Square One Publishers, 2005.

Dossey, Larry. *Space, Time, & Medicine*. Boulder, Shambhala, 1982.

Eisenberg, Arlene. *What to Expect When You're Expecting*. New York, Workman Publishing, 1991.

Epstein, Gerald. *Healing into Immortality: a New Spiritual Medicine of Healing Stories and Imagery*. New York, Bantam Books, 1994.

Erickson, Milton H. *My Voice Will Go with You: The Teaching Tales of Milton H. Erickson*. Ed. Sidney Rosen. New York: Norton, 1982.

Erickson, Milton H., and Jeffrey K. Zeig. *Teaching Seminar with Milton H. Erickson, M.D.* New York, Brunner/Mazel, 1980.

Faber, Adele et al. *How to Talk so Kids Will Listen & Listen so Kids Will Talk*. New York, NY, Scribner Classics, 2012.

Feintuch, Stacey. "Rocky Road: Working on Your Marriage When Your Child Has Special Needs." *New Jersey Family*, Sept. 2016.

Feldenkrais, Moshe. *Body and Mature Behavior: A Study of Anxiety, Sex, Gravitation, and Learning*. New York: International Universities, 1950.

Feldenkrais, Moshe, and Michaeleen Kimmey. *The Potent Self: the Dynamics of the Body and the Mind*. Berkeley, CA, Frog, 2003.

Feldenkrais, Moshe, and Thomas Hanna. *Explorers of Humankind*. San Francisco, Harper & Row, 1979.

Feldenkrais, Moshe. *Awareness through Movement: Health Exercises for Personal Growth / Moshe Feldenkrais*. 1990.

Feldenkrais, Moshe. *Body Awareness as Healing Therapy: the Case of Nora*. Berkeley, CA, North Atlantic Books/Frog, 1993.

Feuerstein, Georg, and Stephan Bodian. *Living Yoga: a Comprehensive Guide for Daily Life*. New York, NY, J.P. Tarcher/Perigee, 1993.

Frymann, Viola M., and Hollis H. King. *Proceedings of the International Research Conference Celebrating the 20th Anniversary of the Osteopathic Center for Children*. Indianapolis, IN, American Academy of Osteopathy, 2005.

Frymann, Viola M., and Hollis Heaton. King. *The Collected Papers of Viola M. Frymann: Legacy of Osteopathy to Children*. Indianapolis, IN, The Academy, 1998.

Frymann, Viola M. et al. "Effect of Osteopathic Medical Management on Neurologic Development in Children." *Journal of Association of Osteopathic Medicine*, vol. 92, no. 6, June 1992.

Frymann, Viola M. "Expanding the Osteopathic Concept." *Student Doctor*, vol. 11, no. 3.

Frymann, Viola M. "The Whole Patient Needs A Whole Physician." *Journal of Holistic Medicine*, vol. 2, no. 1, 1992.

Geralis, Elaine. *Children with Cerebral Palsy: a Parent's Guide.* Bethesda, MD, Woodbine House, 1998.

Glazov, Gregory Yuri. *The Bridling of the Tongue and the Opening of the Mouth in Biblical Prophecy.* Sheffield, England, Sheffield Academic Press, 2001.

Goodrich, Janet. *How to Improve Your Child's Eyesight Naturally: A Thoughtful Parent's Guide.* N.p.: Healing Arts, 2004.

Gopnik, Alison. *The Gardener and the Carpenter: What the New Science of Child Development Tells Us about the Relationship between Parents and Children.* New York, Farrar, Straus and Giroux, 2016.

Guinness, Alma E., editor. *Family Guide to Natural Medicine: How to Stay Healthy the Natural Way.* Pleasantville, NY, Reader's Digest Association, 1993.

Hahnemann, Samuel. *Organon of Medicine.* Los Angeles, J.P. Tarcher, 1982.

Hanna, Thomas. *Somatics: Reawakening the Mind's Control of Movement, Flexibility, and Health.* Cambridge, MA, Da Capo, 2004.

Haley, Jay. *Uncommon Therapy: The Psychiatric Techniques of Milton H. Erickson, M.D.* New York: Norton, 1973.

Horrigan, Bonnie. "Jim Jealous, DO: Healing and the Natural World." *Alternative Therapies*, vol. 3, no. 1, Jan. 1997.

Howard, Jane. *Margaret Mead, a Life.* New York: Simon and Schuster, 1984.

Ingall, Marjorie. *Mamaleh Knows Best: What Jewish Mothers Do to Raise Successful, Creative, Empathetic, Independent Children.* New York, Harmony Books, 2016.

Iyengar, B.K.S., and Kofi Busia. *Iyengar: the Yoga Master.* Boston, Shambhala, 2007.

Iyengar, B.K.S. *Astada YogaMala: Collected Works.* Vol. 1-6. New Delhi, Mumbai: Allied Private, 2006.

Iyengar, B.K.S. *Astadala Yogamala: Collected Works (vols. 4-6).* New Delhi, Allied Publishers, 2000.

Iyengar, B.K.S. *Commemoration Volume: 70 Glorious Years of Yogacharya.* Bombay: Light on Yoga Research Trust, 1990.

Iyengar, B.K.S. *Light on Yoga: Yoga Dipika.* New York: Schocken, 1979.

Iyengar, B.K.S. et al. *Light on Life: the Journey to Wholeness, Inner Peace and Ultimate Freedom.* London, Rodale, 2005.

Iyengar, B.K.S. *Yoga: the Path to Holistic Health.* London, Dorling Kindersley Publishers, 2001.

Kavner, Richard S., and Lorraine Dusky. *Total Vision.* New York, A & W Publishers, 1978.

Keirsey, David, and Marilyn M. Bates. *Please Understand Me: Character & Temperament Types*. Del Mar, CA, Distributed by Prometheus Nemesis Book Co., 1984.

Koetzsch, Ronald E. *The Parents' Guide to Alternatives in Education*. Boston, Shambhala, 1997.

Konnikova, Maria. "How People Learn to Become Resilient." *The New Yorker*, The New Yorker, 5 Oct. 2016, http://www.newyorker.com/science/maria-konnikova/the-secret-formula-for-resilience.

Leach, Penelope. *Your Baby & Child: From Birth to Age Five*. London: Alfred A. Knopf, 2010.

Levine, Melvin D. *Keeping a Head in School: a Student's Book about Learning Abilities and Learning Disorders*. Cambridge, MA, Educators Publishing Service, 1990.

Lobato, Debra J. *Brothers, Sisters, and Special Needs: Information and Activities for Helping Young Siblings of Children with Chronic Illnesses and Developmental Disabilities*. Baltimore, P.H. Brookes Publishing Co., 1990.

Lodewyks, Michelle R. "Strength in Diversity: Positive Impacts of Children with Disabilities." *The Vanier Institute of the Family*, The Vanier Institute, 2016, vanierinstitute.ca/children-disability-positive-impacts-children-family/.

Mackinnon, Kate. *From My Hands and Heart: Achieving Health and Balance with Craniosacral Therapy*. Carlsbad, CA, Hay House, Inc., 2013.

Marshak, Laura E., and Fran Prezant. *Married with Special-Needs Children: a Couples' Guide to Keeping Connected*. Bethesda, MD, Woodbine House, 2007.

Mates-Youngman, Kathleen. *Couples Therapy Workbook: 30 Guided Conversations to Re-Connect Relationships*. Eau Claire, WI, Pesi Publishing & Media, 2014.

Mead, Margaret. *Coming of Age in Samoa: A Psychological Study of Primitive Youth for Western Civilisation*. New York: W. Morrow, 1928.

Meyer, Donald J. *The Sibling Slam Book: What It's Really like to Have a Brother or Sister with Special Needs*. Bethesda, MD, Woodbine House, 2005.

Meyer, Donald J. *Views from Our Shoes: Growing up with a Brother or Sister with Special Needs*. Bethesda, MD, Woodbine House, 1997.

Montagu, Ashley. *Touching: the Human Significance of the Skin*. New York, Columbia University Press, 1971.

Moore, Cory et al. *A Reader's Guide for Parents of Children with Mental, Physical, or Emotional Disabilities*. Rockville, MD, U.S. Dept. of Health, Education, and Welfare, Public Health Service, Health Services Administration, Bureau of Community Health Services, 1976.

Morgan, Peggy Lou. *Parenting an Adult With Disabilities or Special Needs: Everything You Need to Know to Plan for and Protect Your Child's Future*. Amacom, 2009.

Myers, Isabel Briggs, and Peter B. Myers. *Gifts Differing: Understanding Personality Type*. Palo Alto, CA, Davies-Black Publishing, 1995.

Nongard, Richard K. *Speak Ericksonian: Mastering the Hypnotic Methods of Milton Erickson*. N.p.: Peachtree Professional Education, 2014.

O'Toole, Donna R. *Facing Change: Falling Apart and Coming Together Again in the Teen Years; a Book about Loss and Change for Teens*. Burnsville, NC, Mountain Rainbow Publications, 1995.

Pueschel, Siegfried M. *The Special Child: a Source Book for Parents of Children with Developmental Disabilities*. Baltimore, Paul H. Brookes Publishing, 1995.

Rando, Therese A. *Grief, Dying, and Death: Clinical Interventions for Caregivers*. Champaign, IL, Research Press Co., 1984.

Rando, Therese A. *How to Go on Living When Someone You Love Dies*. New York, Bantam Books, 1991.

Rando, Therese A. *Loss and Anticipatory Grief*. Lexington, MA, Lexington Books, 1986.

Rando, Therese A. *Treatment of Complicated Mourning*. Champaign, IL, Research Press, 1993.

Rosenfeld, Albert. "Teaching the Body How to Program the Brain Is Moshe's 'Miracle.'" *Smithsonian Magazine*, Jan. 1981.

Rogers, Fred. *The World According to Mr. Rogers: Important Things to Remember*. New York, NY, Hyperion, 2003.

Ross, Alan O. *The Exceptional Child in the Family; Helping Parents of Exceptional Children*. New York, Grune & Stratton, 1964.

Sacks, Oliver. *A Leg to Stand On*. New York, Summit Books, 1984.

Safer, Jeanne. *The Normal One: Life with a Difficult or Damaged Sibling*. New York, Bantam Dell, 2003.

Salzberg, Sharon. *Real Happiness: the Power of Meditation: a 28-Day Program*. New York, Workman Publishing, 2011.

Sandler, Stephen. *New Way to Health: a Guide to Osteopathy*. London, Hamlyn, 1989.

Sandler, Stephen. *Osteopathy and Obstetrics*. Tunbridge Wells, Kent, Anshan, 2012.

Sanford, Matthew. *Waking: a Memoir of Trauma and Transcendence*. Emmaus, PA, Rodale, 2006.

Sanford, Matthew. *Waking: a Passage into Body*. Emmaus, PA, Rodale, 2006.

Solomon, Andrew. *Far from the Tree: Parents, Children and the Search for Identity*. New York, Scribner, 2012.

Speads, Carola H. *Breathing: the ABC's*. New York, Harper & Row, 1978.

Speads, Carola H. *Ways to Better Breathing*. Rochester, VT, Healing Arts Press, 1992.

Steenbarger, Brett. "Two Powerful Reasons to Keep a Journal." *Forbes*, Forbes Magazine, 10 July 2015, www.forbes.com/sites/brettsteenbarger/2015/07/10/two-powerful-reasons-to-keep-a-journal/ #2f038f6d4.

Stough, Carl, and Reece Stough. *Dr. Breath: the Story of Breathing Coordination*. New York, Morrow, 1970.

Sumar, Sonia. *Yoga for the Special Child: a Therapeutic Approach for Infants and Children with Down Syndrome, Cerebral Palsy, and Learning Disabilities*. Buckingham, VA, Special Yoga Publications, 1997.

Sutherland, William G. *The Cranial Bowl; a Treatise Relating to Cranial Articular Mobility, Cranial Articular Lesions and Cranial Technic.* Mankato, MN, Free Press Company, 1939.

Swift, Sally. *Centered Riding.* London, J.A. Allen, 2006.

Tough, Paul. *Helping Children Succeed: What Works and Why.* Boston, Houghton Mifflin Harcourt, 2016.

Tough, Paul. *How Children Succeed: Grit, Curiosity, and the Hidden Power of Character.* Boston, Houghton Mifflin Harcourt, 2012.

Weil, Andrew. *Health and Healing: Understanding Conventional and Alternative Medicine.* Boston, Houghton Mifflin, 1983.

Wildman, Frank. "The Feldenkrais Method: Clinical Applications." *Physical Therapy Forum*, 19 Feb. 1986.

Woodham, Anne, and David Peters. *DK Encyclopedia of Healing Therapies.* London, DK Publishing, 1997.

Wright, Hal. *The Complete Guide to Creating a Special Needs Life Plan: a Comprehensive Approach Integrating Life, Resource, Financial, and Legal Planning to Ensure a Brighter Future for a Person with a Disability.* London, Jessica Kingsley Publishers, 2013.

Zieg, Jeffrey K., ed. *A Teaching Seminar with Milton Erickson.* New York: Brunner/Mazel, 1980.

Zukav, Gary. *The Seat of the Soul.* New York: Simon and Schuster, 1999.

INDEX

ACKNOWLEDGMENTS

Many people assisted and supported me during the writing of this book and no one more than Christine Corso, who guided, edited, revised, and researched—whose belief in me made this book possible. This book is a product of her wisdom and generosity and her collaboration. Thank you Vincent Corso and Jean Mizutani for your substantial contributions and James Rattazzi for patience, positivity, and genius. Thanks to Lori Podvesker for making a bridge for me. Claire Keerl inspired. Suzanna "Neely" Yates, "digital native," taught me to be tech savvy beyond my wildest imagination, and thank you to Julia Corso who helped to bring it home. Phyllis Zilkha, PhD. put "the icing on the cake" and kept me on track. Thank you to my teachers who over forty-five years have imparted their knowledge with insight, wit, and grace. Thank you to the teacher of my teachers, BKS Iyengar, whose wisdom is the foundation of my search for knowledge and meaning. Thank you to Dr. Viola Frymann for her brilliance and sharing the light of it. My family was enthusiastic and kept faith in me. For my husband, Jay, I have no words to express my gratitude and love.

AUTHOR BIO

Laura Shapiro Kramer currently lives on Cape Cod. To learn more about her and read her essays "Can You Show Me Tomorrow Today?" visit UncommonVoyage.com.